a social history of helping services

a social history of helping services

clinic, court, school, and community

murray levine
and
adeline levine
state university of new york at buffalo

a social history of helping services

clinic, court, school, and community

murray levine
and
adeline levine
state university of new york at buffalo

APPLETON-CENTURY-CROFTS
Educational Division
MEREDITH CORPORATION

New York

to David, Zachary, and our other colleagues

contents

acknowledgments

Through their support and interest, our colleagues at the Yale Psycho-Educational Clinic have helped us to write this book. We owe a special debt to Seymour B. Sarason, who first brought the necessity for historical studies to our attention, who shared ideas with us, read and commented on earlier drafts of all the chapters, and who allocated some of the resources of the clinic to this work. Without his interest and encouragement, this work would not have been undertaken, much less completed.

We are also very much indebted to a number of other people who graciously granted interviews, or who read and criticized various chapters. These people include E. K. Wickman, George S. Stevenson, Everett S. Rademacher, David Levy, and Milton Senn, who all contributed to the chapter on the child guidance clinics. Morris Viteles was helpful in shaping the discussion of Witmer. Rube Borough and Charles Larsen were among many who contributed to the chapter on Ben Lindsey. Staughton Lynd read much of the manuscript, ostensibly to check historical fidelity, but he also offered some rather keen psychological observations which were most helpful. Other friends and colleagues who read through and commented upon a goodly portion of earlier drafts include Barbara Frankel, Janet Rosenberg, Marcia Guttentag, and Paul Weiss.

Our sons, David and Zachary, deserve special mention and commendation for participating with their parents in this work for a good part of the last several years. "When you can't lick 'em, join 'em" must have been their motto, for they joined in making the book almost a family project. They also contributed a great many potential titles, all of which were wittier, if less descriptive, than the one we finally selected for the book.

The following publishers kindly granted us permission to quote from copyrighted works. The specific quotations are identified in the text.

> American Journal of Orthopsychiatry
> Appleton-Century-Crofts
> Commonwealth Fund
> Little, Brown Company
> Horace Liveright Publishers
> Macmillan Company
> New York Public Education Association
> The Psychological Clinic (Morris Viteles, Ed.)
> Russell Sage Foundation

We also acknowledge our indebtedness to the original authors of material now in the public domain, upon which we relied heavily. This includes the anonymous letter to Jane Addams, first published by Christopher Lasch in his volume *The Social Thought of Jane Addams* (Bobbs-Merrill, 1965). The specific quotations are acknowledged in the text and in the bibliography.

We owe another special debt to Anita Miller, who in this instance was not only secretary, but also research assistant, private eye, locator of missing persons, and cheering section. That the manuscript was completed in good style is due in no small measure to her intelligence, her energy, her capacity for work, and her general good will.

M.L.
A.L.

foreword

American psychology, particularly in the clinical and social areas, has tended to be ahistorical in orientation. A story may here be instructive. Twenty years ago our department was visited for purposes of evaluation by an outside committee of psychologists representing The American Psychological Association. A member of the committee was interviewing one of the graduate students and in the course of the interview he asked the student: "Did you ever read Kohler's *The Mentality of Apes?*" Without batting an eyelash the student replied, "No one reads that anymore. That's old hat." It is my opinion that both then and now the student's reply was not uncharacteristic of the prevailing attitude toward those who came before us—an attitude not peculiar to a particular university.

I have no desire to glamorize the past or to characterize it as a fathomless goldmine. But I certainly do not buy the implicit judgment in American psychology that wisdom is a current commodity which, unfortunately for them, those who came before us could not savor. The scholarly pursuit of the past is not an activity which we ask our students to value highly. They may do an experiment for a thesis, or a correlational study, or, less likely, a series of case studies—but not a scholarly examination of some aspect of the past. When in the mid-thirties Howard Spoerl at Harvard was permitted to do a thesis on Gall and Spurzheim the news spread quickly (psychology was much smaller then!) because it was precedent shattering. But the precedent was far weaker than the tradition and the royal road (narrow and one-way) to human knowledge and understanding was quickly repaved with what the architects of theory building call hard data. If the scholarly pursuit of the past is not made easy for our students, one must say that it is somewhat easier for faculty people, although such pursuit does not give one as many brownie points toward promotion as do the more conventional ways of enlarging a curriculum vita.

The basic issue, however, does not concern the past or present but rather the constriction of the things about which we are or should be curious. What is worrisome is not that our curiosity about the past is blunted but that the value judgments which give rise to such blunting tend not to be made explicit and therefore, discussable in no-holds-barred discussions. I would maintain that when a field is not seriously interested in its past one should hold it as suspect as one would an individual who strenuously avoids thinking about or coming to grips with his past.

When I talk of the past I do not mean the history of a particular problem but rather the changing relationships between a field or subfield, on the one hand, and the societal context in which they are embedded, on the other hand. We like to think that the status of any scientific field is independent of the larger social context, i.e., that theories, methodologies, and problems are only the reflection of the minds and efforts of individual investigators. This unrealistic thinking cannot be scrutinized or evaluated when a field of endeavor does not value highly scholarly investigations of its past relationships to its society.

The preceding paragraphs were not written for polemical purposes but rather to indicate why I value the present book so highly. What the Levines have done is to search the past for what it might tell us about a set of problems with which an increasing number of professionals are currently concerned. I refer here to the conglomerate of problems, issues, and methodologies contained in the unrevealing label of community mental health. After reading the current literature one might justifiably conclude that this is a newly "discovered" field, i.e., it is not only a reaction against the domination over the past several decades of interpersonal theories and techniques, but it also represents a qualitative change in ways of thinking and acting. What this book demonstrates is that this "new" field may be new to *us* but it was truly old hat to a variety of individuals who lived decades ago. This in itself should temper our tendency to assume without questioning that every decade in every way we come to possess new and better knowledge.

But what may be humbling here should also be (as the authors indicate) a source of renewed respect for what man is, has been, and could be. What the reader will find in this book are the accomplishments of some heroic figures who both reflected and transcended their times.

There is one regularity which the Levines discuss in several places in this book, a regularity from which the professional person may not derive satisfaction but which, if faced squarely, may discernibly act as a preventive against the disease of professional preciousness. Stated most simply the regularity goes this way: when a new, creative, and productive combination of ideas and practice become professionalized and institutionalized, the chances are very great that both the form and substance of this combination of ideas and practice become changed beyond recognition. In the end there is the word, whereas at the beginning there was the idea. The Levines help us recapture the idea.

Seymour B. Sarason

Psycho-Educational Clinic
Yale University

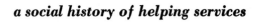
a social history of helping services

1
introduction

We began looking into the early history of clinical problems and clinical services for children out of nothing more than idle curiosity. However, it quickly became apparent that the early history of clinical services for children had great pertinence for the contemporary community mental health movement. While everyone knows that Lightner Witmer started the first psychological clinic in 1896, and that William Healy started the first "real" psychiatric clinic for children in 1909 as part of the Juvenile Court in Chicago, it was not until we started reading the original material that we could find reference to what these early clinics actually did. It was all too easy to assume that early clinics were unsophisticated versions of contemporary clinics, and to dismiss them as having no contemporary relevance. However, as soon as we began our research, we knew we had tapped a rich vein indeed.

Those early services were embedded in the community, were concerned with the educational process, and were oriented toward prevention. In short, the models of clinical services, developed between 1896 and the mid-1920's, demand close examination precisely because our predecessors began with the types of services the community mental health movement seems to be struggling toward today. It was quite a shock to discover that Yale's Psycho-Educational Clinic, established in 1963 as an innovation in clinical services, was somewhat of a throwback to the 1890's!

We were not alone in our innocence. In the spring of 1966, one of us participated in a panel discussion on the relationship between day care centers specializing in educational programming for emotionally disturbed children and public school settings. The panelists presented therapeutic and educational programs which had originated over the last few years. They were rightly concerned with the variation in method from standard psychotherapeutic approaches and with evaluating their own approaches. However, none of the panelists had any awareness that Witmer had developed clinic teaching as a therapeutic approach, that he had regular classes conducted as part of his clinic, that he had developed a hospital school, and that he had consciously concerned himself with the problem of transferring gains made in the clinic to the public school setting. Similarly, none of the panelists was aware that the Commonwealth Demonstration Clinics of the mid-1920's were developed concomitant with an effort to promote the visiting teacher movement, and that considerable effort was made to try to integrate the work of clinics with the work of the public schools. The problems that the 1966 workers were discussing bore an amazing similarity to those faced by workers several generations earlier, but they were being approached as if they were brand new.

It is a regrettable tendency of our field to neglect the history of research problems. We adopt the physical science model with its assumption that earlier knowledge is fully incorporated into the most recent theory and technology. We search the abstracts for the last ten years, and generally do not go back any further; we seem to say that no worthwhile work could possibly have been forgotten that was done in the past. A personal example will illustrate the point. Some years ago one of us was engaged in research which revealed a small but significant correlation between measures of sensory sensitivity and intelligence. It was not until long afterwards that we discovered this was a path traversed by pre-Binet researchers in the field, and abandoned as unfruitful because of the meagerness and inconsistency of findings in the area. In retrospect there was nothing to suggest that we would do any better following that particular lead than did Galton, Cattell, or Whipple. Had we been aware of that early literature, our own research probably would have taken a different turn.

We use this story to illustrate Santayana's well-known maxim that those who forget the past are doomed to repeat it. For the social scientist, the maxim provides a succinct comment on deficiencies in his methods of studying every kind of human behavior. It is our newly found feeling that most of those social problems which fall within the province of the social sciences do recur in similar form, in different places, and at different times, and probably for quite similar reasons.

In the present instance, there is much to be learned because the models and the experiences of the past are relevant. There are ideas and practices which should be recovered precisely because mental health professionals are going into the same fields, and are unwittingly using modes of approach very similar to those of the past.

There is another reason for examining the past. The early services started out with what we would today call a community orientation, and a preventive orientation, but in the course of a relatively few years, the services changed. Where Witmer's clinic was closely involved with the public schools, and where the Commonwealth clinics of the 1920's made a conscious effort to relate to the public schools, it is commonplace today that child guidance clinics have either no contact or minimal contact with the teachers and principals of children they treat. Just a few months ago, one of us working in the schools had occasion to inquire about a child new to the school who was under treatment at a child guidance clinic. The treating psychiatrist felt free in sharing information with us, but he had no knowledge whatsoever about what the child's behavior had been like in school. He had not seen it as part of his function. We do not cite this example to criticize a psychiatrist, but merely to point out how radically practices have changed over the years.

The contemporary child guidance clinic is professionally staffed, and offers individual, group, or family psychotherapy, and intake and diagnostic services. Most clinics have a rather small investment in consultation with community agencies or with schools. A very small proportion of clinic time is spent in community education, and we would venture to guess that virtually no time at all is spent in attempting to influence local and state government to improve social conditions which cause or exacerbate given mental health problems. Clinics operate on the medical model of treating those who voluntarily bring themselves to the clinic, and they do not ordinarily seek out cases. Preventive thinking is barely beginning to come into its own right at the present time.

In the perspective of history, contemporary clinical services for children, as described above, are a failure. The fact that any treatment oriented in-clinic service would be immediately swamped was apparent from the earliest days, and the early clinics consciously intended to avoid getting bogged down in a treatment load. However, they quickly developed discouragingly long waiting lists. They intended to develop preventive modes of help, but here, too, they were unsuccessful. Witmer's clinic, Healy's clinic, the visiting teacher movement, the settlement houses, and the early Commonwealth Fund Demonstration Clinics were closely tied in with a variety of community agencies. Contemporary clinics are not, as a general rule. The goal of influencing those in the natural setting to care for mental health problems more effectively, a goal the early clinics had, had been carried through only to the limited extent that psychiatric teaching influenced the development of professional social work, but even this influence has been limited. The graduate schools of social work turn out a pitifully small number of trained workers each year. A great number of these workers function as psychotherapists and have limited social influence.

This phenomenon of change in clinical services demands study. There are reasons for changes in practice. One of the viewpoints we will try to develop is that change is as much due to a variety of social forces as it is due to well-supported developments in the science of human behavior. It is our argument that it is necessary to pay attention to the larger social and historical context of the development of various services in order to understand why certain services developed and why they changed.

Our examination of the history of the field will show that many of the most creative innovations in practice were initiated and carried through by people who were outside the professional mental health fields. The early settlement house workers were responsible in part for the establishment of the Juvenile Court, with its system of probation workers, and the first probation worker was the very model of the indigenous nonprofessional. The court was operating effectively as a helping agency for ten years before the psychiatrist William Healy began his work with it. The settlement house workers also originated the visiting teacher concept, the forerunner of the school social worker. Judge Ben Lindsey, who developed the Juvenile Court in Denver, had a concept of the court of law as an institute of human relations whose function it was to help people and not punish them. Lindsey, noted for his contributions in law, and later notorious for his advocacy of companionate marriage, has been forgotten as a clinician, although his therapeutic achievements and his methods reflected a human artistry of the highest form. Nor should we forget that Witmer, trained as an experimental and not as a clinical psychologist, frequently used school teachers in therapeutic roles, and in at least one of the cases he reports, it is perfectly clear that the important therapeutic work was done, with his knowledge and encouragement, by a housemaid. The clinic associated with the Cincinnati Court (circa 1914) made extensive use of volunteers from the Big Brothers, the Rotary, and other civic organizations to work with children who needed help. The child guidance movement itself owes its existence to Clifford Beers. Beers, a Yale graduate and a layman in the field, underwent a severe psychosis. After he recovered, Beers organized the National Committee for Mental Hygiene (1909), and it was this group which pressed for the development of child guidance clinics as preventive agents.

Mental health personnel tend to suffer with what Sarason et al. (1966) have termed "professional preciousness." Preciousness is an attitude which holds that one's professional training has uniquely fitted one for carrying out mental health services, and that anyone who does not have the requisite training not only will not be able to perform such services, but will in fact do harm. It is this attitude which resists innovation in practice, and which is highly sensitive to infringements on roles and functions in any clinical setting. But the contemporary mental health professional is a Johnny-come-lately in a field largely developed by those who were in no way trained for the tasks they performed. Such knowledge provides a basis for humility, and may help us to understand that modes of practice do not necessarily arise as direct consequences of advances in science.

The fact that services originated with non-professionals emphasizes the desirability of studying the social context of the development of those services. They did not originate as conscious extensions of scientific hypotheses, and if they did originate in response to social need, then the services must indeed reflect their times.

We have no intention of producing a comprehensive and detailed history of mental health and social services. Our intent has been to deal selectively with services for children, services which largely originated in the period roughly between 1890 and the mid-1920's. The era from about 1890 to the First World War is one well demarcated period, and the decade from 1920 to 1930 is another. They represent respectively a period of reform and of conservatism, and the change from the one to the other can be seen in the philosophy and imple-mentation of services developed in the two periods. We focused on services for children because that happens to be our primary profes-sional interest at present. There is nothing in the thesis we have developed which restricts itself to specific time periods, or to work with children. In fact, we would suggest that those with an interest in socio-historical research might examine other well-marked periods of change and conservatism to determine whether the principles we have specified will hold for other kinds of helping agencies, and in other ages. Grob's (1966) excellent study of the state mental hospital in the mid-19th century is a case in point.

We are amateur historians who have ventured into an area where we have little expertise. We are trained in the methods of quantitatively oriented experimental social science, and have little knowledge of the methods of hypothesis testing used by historians or social philosophers. However, we have been greatly impressed by the potential in historical study for elucidating socio-psychological theory, and for providing, if not hard data and quantitatively tested and testable generalizations, then lessons, parallels, analogues, or models which can be used in understanding the present, and even in making predictions to the future. While testimonials and unverified claims based upon personal experience do not constitute the stuff of science, we do not hesitate to assert that our own clinical work with low-income groups has been much enhanced by our new-found historical perspective. While there are undoubtedly differences in the present, the problems poor urban residents had around the turn of the century, and the difficulties helping agencies had then in attempting to deal with the problems are strikingly similar to the problems and difficulties encountered today. In fact, it is our feeling that some of the difficulties plaguing anti-poverty programs today might have been predicted and avoided had their designers paid serious attention to social history.

It is this sense of the power of the historical study of social processes which has stimulated an introspective concern with our research method. There are some numbers in this book, but quantities are used illustratively and not as indices which test hypotheses. We have neither sampled nor attempted to be comprehensive in our discussion of people, periods, and programs. The picture emerged for us as we got into the material, and as we traced down various programs. As Carr (1961) suggests in his methodology of history, the process of writing history is a process of telling a coherent story. We may have created a more coherent picture than the material warranted by imposing ourselves on what we chose to consider and to present. However, we retain a conviction that the view we present is a workable reconstruction of reality, arrived at by a process of examining evidence, and testing theory against evidence. While we are not in a position to formalize a statement of method, we agree with Dollard (1957), who argues that "The primary research instrument would seem to be the observing human intelligence trying to make sense out of experience" (p. 18). We do wish to assert our belief that formal methodology ought to be developed to make it possible to deal systematically in the empirically oriented social sciences with historical data, without totally reducing the sweep of history to pedantic and obsessional counts of words or phrases.

The most important events are those which usually cannot be studied as they occur nor can they be created in all their vitality and complexity in any laboratory. Moreover, significant human events often take place over time periods which do not meet the researcher's academic-year limitations. If method is to be adapted to the problem, and not the other way around, then it may be that historical study, viewing events in the context of their time, and in the perspective offered by temporal distance, is a major way of dealing with socio-psychological issues. If so, the approach needs its own philosophy of method. The methods of control, the definition of the conditions of observation, and limitations on the inferences and generalizations which can be drawn from any set of observations need to be developed with due consideration for the nature of human documents and historical study. Our present approach may have more kinship with that of the artist or the historical novelist than with the quantitative empiricist, but it is our feeling as social scientists that the material demands such an approach. We feel intuitively that it is worthwhile to try to tell a coherent story even if we do not count the number of positive and negative instances found in some sample of documents in the time period of interest. With Jules Henry (1965), we are as interested in events which occurred often enough to be noticed and recorded as we are in how often the events occurred. Perhaps it is our professional conscience which leads us to warn others about how we undertook this project, but we also feel a regret that our own scientific training did not prepare us in any way to deal confidently with historical data.

Our purposes then in writing this book are several. First, it is our intent simply to describe a variety of helping services and the conditions under which they developed. We want to call attention to certain modes of operation, and the problems earlier workers encountered in order that we neither blindly repeat the past, nor obtusely lose valuable models.

Second, it is the purpose of this book to explore the thesis that social and economic conditions and the intellectual and political spirit of the times exert profound influences upon the particular mental health problems which concern us and upon the particular forms of help which develop and flourish. As a corollary of this thesis one can argue that changes in the forms of help are shaped at least as much by the predominant social forces of the times as they are by thoroughly supported developments in the science of human behavior.

More specifically, the thesis states there are essentially two modes of help, the situational and the intra-psychic. The situational mode assumes a person who is basically "good" but who has been exposed to poor conditions, and therefore has not developed to his fullest potential. Improving his situation will result in far-reaching improvement in his psychological state. The intra-psychic mode assumes a person who is in difficulty, not because of his situation, but because of his inner weaknesses and failings; it assumes the situation is more or less irrelevant, that what has to be changed is not the circumstance but the person.

The present thesis argues that situational modes of help, demanding as they do the questioning of the social environment and change in the social environment, will flourish during periods of political or social reform, periods we now believe are better described by the term "acute social change." Then society is ready for change, and will accept change. Intra-psychic modes of help, focusing as they do on the inadequacies of the individual, assume the "goodness" of the environment. Intra-psychic modes of help will be prominent during periods of political or social conservatism, for the intra-psychic mode tends to support the status quo by placing the onus of both the problem and the change on the mind and emotions of the individual. We cannot claim originality for this thesis. Cohen (1958) mentions a similar viewpoint briefly in his history of American social work. However, the present elaboration of the thesis is our responsibility.

It should be clear that no one period will be exclusively dominated by one or another form of help, and that each period will be marked by an intermingling of both forms of help. Each reform period has conservative critics, just as each conservative period has reform critics. Each period contains the seeds for the dominant form of the next period, so that we cannot expect unambiguous support for the thesis at any point in time.

While the hypothesis itself is not readily amenable to empirical test, it is the sort of hypothesis which serves to direct attention to observations which themselves may become clear only in historical perspective. It is an hypothesis which has value in the present and in the immediate future because it directs attention to variables mental health professionals ordinarily ignore. At this time, when the mental health professional is moving out into the community, he is well advised to be aware of how political and social realities limit and shape his potential for action. The hypothesis was formulated and stated, just as this historical study was undertaken, because of its relevance today.

2

the climate of change

The field of mental health is currently in a state of ferment so strong that some have already termed the present period the beginning of its third major revolution. The first revolution dates from the time that Pinel removed the chains from mental patients, insisting they were sick and not sinful. The second revolution dates from Freud's introduction of psychodynamic concepts. The third revolution, which refers to the community mental health movement, is probably best dated by President Kennedy's address to Congress in 1963 in which he called for a radically new approach to the care of the mentally ill.

The radically new approach not only involves the *reintegration* of recovered mental patients into the community; it also involves the *prevention* of the personal waste and misery we term mental, emotional, or behavioral disorder, and the promotion of positive mental health. Positive mental health means more than the absence of symptoms. It means that state of well-being which enables the individual to pursue his personal fulfillment. These are bold and broad objectives for community mental health programs, for as soon as the field deals with concepts of positive mental health, the mental health professional must concern himself with studying and influencing those major institutions of society which create, perpetuate, or exacerbate personal waste and misery. In a sense, the whole quality of American life becomes his concern. The mental health professional retains his interest in the individual who is in distress, but in his role as helper he wishes also to influence the family, the schools, social agencies, the courts, industrial organization, community life, the legal and governmental structure, and the economic order. His role model changes from that of the physician and healer to that of educator, social critic, reformer, and social planner.

The contemporary community mental health movement must also be considered from the perspective of its place in American society. Its broad goals must be viewed as a product of the growing acceptance by American society for the total welfare of all individuals. The contemporary period reflects the trends which began with the industrial revolution, which were accelerated with the rapid social changes induced by processes of industrialization and urbanization, and which continue today, powered by scientific and technical developments. Throughout our history, but particularly from the 1870's onward, the responsibility of government for the welfare of the people has become increasingly clear and increasingly pervasive. President Johnson spoke as a matter of national policy of the attainment of the Great Society, in which each individual would be freed of concern for material survival and enabled to achieve personal fulfillment.

In the mental health field, the change in the concept of governmental responsibility may be seen in the fate of federal legislation relating to the care of the mentally ill. In 1854, President Franklin Pierce (Pierce, 1854) vetoed Dorothea Dix's bill to obtain a federally supported mental hospital on the grounds that the life conditions of individuals were no proper concern of government. In 1955, 101 years later, Congress appointed the Joint Commission on Mental Illness and Mental Health to study the problem and to make recommendations for federal action. When the Joint Commission recommended a narrow program in mental health to be built around the development and revitalization of the state mental hospital system, President Kennedy called for a completely new approach in which the federal government was to take the lead in the prevention and treatment of mental disorder. Federal support, on an unprecedented scale, was to be made available for the development of comprehensive, interlocking community services and facilities in order to identify and to satisfy a whole range of needs. Help was not to be limited to the provision of institutions which isolate the "repulsive" (to use the Joint Commission's apt, if harsh term) for their protection and for the protection of society. The concept of providing comprehensive services was embodied in the Community Mental Health Centers Act of 1963.[1]

The Joint Commission report (1961) stated what had long been known: that it is completely impossible with current patterns of mental health services to meet the needs of any but a tiny fraction of those who need help for mental and emotional problems. Surveys of adult populations (Veroff et al., 1960; Srole et al., 1962) and surveys of populations of children (White & Harris, 1961) show clearly that a distressingly large percentage of Americans suffer psychological complaints which at a minimum create personal misery, and which at worst are severely disabling. We cannot say that more people are disturbed now than at some former time because we do not have evidence.[2] However, we are certainly aware that the available mental health facilities, and particularly outpatient facilities, are overloaded. Almost every mental health clinic or social agency has a long waiting list. Private help is costly, in limited supply, and tends to be concentrated in a few large, urban centers.

Shortage of people and of facilities, not likely to be overcome by expanded training efforts, is one overriding factor in the mental health field. There is little hope that educational facilities can be expanded to meet more than a small fraction of present and future needs for trained personnel (Albee, 1959). The overloading of present facilities is in part a consequence of the rapid increase in population. However, the near inevitability of shortage of treating personnel was recognized by the Commonwealth Demonstration Clinics in the mid-1920's, so it is clear the problem is a chronic one, and not solely the result of the current population explosion. Shortage, though, is a potent factor in opening the mental health field to change.

We have also become aware that the need is most acute in low-income populations. Surveys (Hollingshead & Redlich, 1958; Srole

[1] This act, which provides general guides for the type of service to be conducted, is singularly devoid of elements which might stimulate creative innovation. There is the distinct danger that the new community mental health center will turn out to be nothing more than the old psychopathic hospital with a few frills. Albee's (1965) evaluation of existing models of community mental health centers—"There is nothing on the inside except the same old performers going through the same old routines"—provides little cause for optimism that these centers will exert any important influence on the way in which people actually live.

[2] Goldhamer and Marshall (1953) have shown that rates of hospitalization for psychosis in the state of Massachusetts have not changed in 100 years.

et al., 1962; Leighton et al., 1963) have indicated that emotional problems are both more frequent and more severe in low-income populations, particularly in areas noted for their social disorganization. Surveys of children indicate much the same (White & Harris, 1961). While there are arguments about the amount of unrecorded delinquency, and about differential enforcement of the law, it seems indisputable that low-income populations produce high rates of crime and delinquency. At another level, Knobloch and Pasamanick (1961) have argued that low-income populations have higher rates of prematurity, problems in pregnancy and birth associated with probable brain damage, and a variety of childhood disturbances including speech, reading, and behavioral disorders. The Coleman report (1967) confirms, on a national level, that low-income groups have educational deficits which presage a disastrous social and economic adjustment for these groups. Recently, Moynihan (1965) and Rainwater (1966) have documented a state of disorganization in lower-class Negro families which will perpetuate a variety of social and psychological problems.

While the need is clearly most acute, helping services reach low-income populations at best sparingly, and at worst ineffectively, or even destructively. For adult patients, Hollingshead and Redlich (1958) have shown clearly that low-income patients are most likely to receive custodial or somatic care, while upper-income patients are most likely to receive more intensive and personalized psychotherapy. Myers and Schaffer (1954) showed a similar phenomenon for patients applying for psychotherapy at an outpatient mental hygiene clinic. Upper-income patients were more likely to be accepted for psychotherapy, and when accepted, were most likely to be assigned to more experienced therapists. Class V patients, the lowest group, were more likely to be refused psychotherapeutic help, and when accepted for treatment, were more likely to be assigned to an inexperienced medical student who was to be at the clinic for a four-week period. In view of the questionable effectiveness of psychotherapeutic procedures, the evidence may reveal only that available services do not reach low-income groups in the same way they do other segments of the population. People may not be treated on the basis of what they need, but on the basis of who they are.

The reports of Furman (1965) and of Harrison et al. (1965) suggest that much the same is true for children seen in child guidance clinics in New York City. Low-income patients are generally underrepresented in clinic populations, and when they appear, they are less likely to receive treatment. When we think of the degree of family disorganization in lower-income Negro groups, when we think of the lower-class person's reluctance to deal with authority, and when we think of the requirements most clinics have that at least one, if not both parents, participate in treatment, it is not surprising that lower-income families are systematically screened out of existing child guidance services.

The Juvenile Courts were created with a broad mandate for child welfare and were among the first institutions to use psychiatric services. Now they rarely have treatment facilities. Social agencies rarely provide significant counseling help to their lower-income clientele. AFDC (Aid to Families of Dependent Children) programs generally supervise the purse strings of their clients but rarely if ever provide more personal interest and help to their families, as May (1964) has shown so movingly. Case reports of problems in the relationship of welfare agencies and the Juvenile Court to low-income populations may be found in Sarason et al. (1966).

The public school, another institution which might provide significant help to lower-income children, also has a dearth of services. Those services available have generally been directed to schools in better neighborhoods, according to Sexton's report (1961). Anti-poverty programs and federal aid to education may begin to reach more schoolchildren. However, established programs have not appeared in either the quantity or the quality which would give rise to an optimistic view of the future.

There is another set of internal professional pressures which have helped to create the climate of change. The most prestigious of the helping methods, psychotherapy, has come under strong attack, not only on the grounds that it does not reach the low-income patient, but also on the grounds that the procedures may be ineffective. Eysenck (1952, 1961) led the attack when he marshalled evidence which challenged psychotherapists to show that their efforts over a period of time produced change any more effectively than no special help or a minimum of help over an equal length of time. Levitt (1957) and Levitt, Beiser, and Robertson (1959) summarized similar evidence for psychotherapeutic work with children. While there are many questions about the basic studies, and while there are many unresolved issues of controls, it is perfectly clear that the burden of proof is upon the psychotherapist to demonstrate that his methods are effective. Serious question of the effectiveness of the helping technique obligates the professional to seek alternatives.

In clinical settings, particularly outpatient settings, we have also become aware that a highly significant number of patients drop out of treatment after relatively few interviews. Tuckman and Lavell (1959) reported an overall dropout rate of 58 percent for patients seen at 11 child guidance clinics in Philadelphia. Similar findings are reported by Furman (1965) for clinics in New York City, and there is an extensive literature on dropouts in therapy with adults (Reiss & Brandt, 1965). Some of these patients may benefit from brief contacts, and some eventually enter treatment elsewhere, but it is clear that a great deal of therapeutic and diagnostic time is wasted time. The careful intake at many outpatient facilities, which results in extensive waiting lists, is paradoxical in light of the high rate of discontinuance of treatment in many centers. Every clinician working in such a setting is painfully aware of the problem at some level, although some tend to justify the situation by arguing that therapeutic methods are effective only with those who demonstrate sufficient motivation to stay with treatment. Nonetheless, the existence of the problem in most outpatient settings must contribute to the professional mental health worker's willingness to reevaluate the nature of the services he is currently offering.

In the field of psychodiagnosis, the projective tests and clinical intuition and judgment have also come in for considerable questioning. In the decade of the 1950's innumerable Ph.D. theses and other researches failed to demonstrate that projective tests were of any significant worth. Much of that work is summarized in Rickers-Ovsiankina (1960), in Murstein (1963), and in Zubin, Eron, and Schumer (1965). Meehl (1954) unleashed a thunderbolt when he demonstrated that the clinician's vaunted clinical intuition was no better, and in many instances much worse, as a predictive device than a simple regression equation based upon standard, mechanical psychometric research. In subsequent years, Meehl (1960) continued his assault upon the clinical, psychodiagnostic enterprise showing that a clinician's appraisal of a case could not effectively influence a therapist's judgment. Therapists arrived at formulations of their cases within a relatively few hours and did not seem to need diagnostic tests after those few hours. While there still may be instances in which diagnostic tests may contribute significantly to decisions about treatment, evidence seems to suggest that a good deal of diagnostic testing is wasted, particularly in view of high dropout rates. There is not one study which shows that therapy was either reduced in length of time or was more effective as a consequence of diagnostic testing. The attack on the psychologist's functions has led to the reconsideration of the role and its clinical significance.

The role of the mental health professional is under pressure to change not only because of the inadequacies of current forms of treatment, but also because recent thinking in the field has suggested that aspects of practice may actually produce more mental health problems than are cured. The Joint Commission's report *Action for Mental Health* (1961) described the overcrowding and understaffing of the large mental hospitals which made for a custodial rather than a therapeutic orientation. Chronicity may be produced and encouraged by efforts to manage patients in the cheapest and most convenient ways in total institutions (Goffman, 1961) which remove the "repulsive" from the community. That society has been more interested in removing deviants from the community than in restoring them to the community is demonstrated in the lag in the development of aftercare services. At the present time, Connecticut, the home state of Clifford Beers and a pioneer in providing aftercare for mental patients, has minimal aftercare services. In New Haven, for example, it has been our experience that patients released from state mental hospitals typically will be seen once a month, if that often, for supervision of medication; more intensive care is almost impossible to obtain. We are not criticizing the quality of care in Connecticut facilities. We are simply using this enlightened state as an example to reveal the very limited aftercare which is available.

Not only is there a problem in finding facilities for aftercare, but a patient who returns after a sojourn in a mental hospital finds himself stigmatized by his community. Partly because of the problems which are caused by the huge state hospitals, the brand-new community mental health centers are experimenting with services and techniques intended to maintain the patient in the community with minimal dislocation in his life and in the lives of his family. Day hospitals, night hospitals, intensive treatment services, emergency care in crises, family therapy, and the inclusion of vocational rehabilitative services with mental hospital care all have as goals the integration of the patient (and the mental hospital) with the immediately surrounding community. The problem of stigma, so well described by Cumming and Cumming (1957; 1965), by Goffman (1963), and by Phillips (1967), is not entirely solved by such measures. Nonetheless, if the patient can be kept at home, and on his job, his reentry problem may be reduced considerably. The experimentation with new services and techniques requires that the mental health professional reorient himself to his role in the hospital and in the community, for he will be less likely to be living and working in the small, closed society of a psychiatric hospital or clinic.

The problem of the adult mental patient has received most of the attention, but no less severe a problem exists in the care of dependent, delinquent, mentally deficient, and mentally ill children. Residential treatment facilities are generally in short supply. The level of care in many of the institutions borders on the scandalous, and in not a few cases the borders have been crossed (Blatt & Kaplan, 1966). There is an increasing demand for residential services for children, but we have yet to see comparable concern about returning children to the community or maintaining them there. In our work with a local anti-poverty agency we have come across instances of adolescents who spent their formative years in institutions with limited academic and vocational facilities, and then were released at age 18 into the community to fend for themselves. After 18, the state no longer had any formal legal responsibility for these boys. The few cases who came to our attention were living an aimless and lonely existence in a shabby midtown hotel. Recognizing the problems in the field of mental deficiency, Connecticut has developed the regional center concept (Sarason et al., 1966). Smaller institutions with a limited number of inpatient beds are located in population centers, with the mission of assisting the local community to maintain most of the retarded children in their own homes.

A still more subtle problem for the mental health field is raised by recent sociological thinking about mental illness as deviancy, and mental health facilities as agencies of deviance control. In this view, most recently explicated by Scheff (1966), psychiatric patients are seen as those who have engaged in what Scheff calls "residual rule-breaking." Residual rule-breaking refers to a variety of violations for which a society provides no explicit label. In our society the violators tend to get lumped together as mentally ill. This viewpoint enables one to consider the behavior called mental illness as bound to "culturally particular normative networks," and not as culture-free symptoms of disease. The social context in which symptoms appear then becomes vital, and the social context and the social norms are open to investigation as contributory to what we call mental illness.

Scheff (1966) argues that almost everyone engages in rule-breaking of various kinds, but only a small percentage of residual rule-breakers go on to deviant careers. That is, in only a very small percentage of the cases does the rule-breaking behavior become stabilized. Scheff wants to account for stabilized residual rule-breaking in terms of the societal reaction to it. The rule-breaking individual is defined as a patient, he takes on that role, and he is then subjected to all of the constraints which act in concert to prevent him from reentering the realm of the normal.

The implications of this view are profound. For one, the mental health professions, and psychiatry in particular, are viewed as contributing to the development of mental illness by providing the doctor role, the necessary complement to the patient role. In effect, by treating a patient in a separate treating institution, the doctor certifies that the patient is indeed a patient and is indeed mentally ill. If the social setting in which the residual rule-breaking occurred had some means of dealing with the problem behavior other than certifying the deviant as ill, the individual would be less likely to enter the sick role, and the deviant behavior would be less likely to stabilize. Community-oriented approaches, in which normal caretakers, policemen, teachers, lawyers, ministers, and the like are encouraged to handle residual rule-breaking by means other than psychiatric referral might obviate considerably the problems of the sick role. A very new function, that of human relations consultant and advisor to the caretaker, is implied for the mental health professional, not only because the numbers problem demands it but because, in the end, it may prove a more effective way of helping.

There is a second implication in this sociological theory of mental illness. The mental health professionals must be viewed as agents of deviance control. Not only is the mental health professional the one who identifies the deviant; in the very doing he confirms the validity of the social norm violated. The mental health professional is accorded a position with considerable status and considerable wealth attached to it, but in turn the mental health professional confirms the norms of the society which rewards him. In periods of relative social stability, there may be little problem in the mental health professional acting to confirm societal norms. However, in periods of acute social change, *the mental health professional may contribute to the exacerbation of the dislocations people endure by becoming part of the process which induces and maintains cultural lag.* The mental health professional may be confirming social norms which no longer have viability in terms of the way in which people actually live in a changing society.

We shall want to develop this viewpoint to a greater extent later. For now, let us say only that the signs that the mental health profession is under pressure to change suggest to us, along with evidence that many other institutions are also under pressure to change (e.g., the schools, the courts, the churches, welfare agencies, patterns of occupations), that contemporary American society is in a period of acute social change. We shall want to speculate about the nature of that change and the new helping forms which we predict will arise in the near future, but only after we have developed the historical base for the theoretical view sketched in the introduction.

The variety of forces we have described—population growth, social disorganization associated with personal misery, and the variety of inadequacies of the current pattern of services to serve that segment of the population with the greatest needs—are all factors currently creating both a climate of openness to change and an intense interest in community mental health. The phrase "community mental health" seems to be new. It seems to stand for a set of concepts and techniques as yet only half-formed. However, in the history of mental health services for children, the ideas defining contemporary concepts of community mental health programs are not new; and in fact they hark back to the very inception of a variety of professional services for children.

As we shall see when we describe the actual operation of early clinical facilities and clinical services, we will be talking about far more than the simple idea that our intellectual progenitors said it first. They not only said it first, but if today a clinic were organized and functioning like the early clinics, it would be hailed as the very model of what a community mental health clinical service ought to be.[3] The Psycho-Educational Clinic program, (Sarason, et al., 1966), which

[3] Compare the activities of the South Shore Clinic, as described by Rosenblum and Ottenstein (1965), with the Child Guidance Clinics of the 1920's (Chapter 9).

developed as a radical departure from contemporary child guidance practice, has much more in common with Witmer's clinic first developed in 1896, with the visiting teacher movement initiated in 1906, and with the Commonwealth Fund Child Guidance Clinics of the mid-1920's than it does with contemporary psychiatric clinics for children, or with case work and family service agencies providing services to children.

The early clinical services for children developed with an orientation toward the community, and then changed directions. An examination of these clinical services and their history will enrich us in several ways. First, there are a number of valuable concepts which can be reexamined profitably in terms of the organization and actual practices of these services. Second, the clinical services changed over the course of time. If contemporary services are to learn anything from those experiences, and if we are to try to predict the future, a close examination of the kinds of changes which took place, and the reasons for the changes is in order. Third, we have stated the general thesis that social and economic conditions and the intellectual and political spirit of the times exert profound influences upon the mental health problems which occupy our attention, and upon the forms of help which develop and change. History can be the proving ground for such a thesis. In the next chapter, the reader will be offered a description of the historical and social conditions under which a variety of children's services developed.

3

1890 - 1914: an era of reform

Almost all modern professional services for children were established in the years between 1890 and the beginning of the First World War as part of a general concern about the welfare of children.[1] Cohen (1958) lists the following agencies which were concerned directly or indirectly with child welfare and with services to children: The Family Service Association (1911); U.S. Children's Bureau (1912); National Committee for Mental Hygiene (1909); the national organization of the YWCA (1906); National Federation of Settlements (1911); Boy Scouts (1910); Camp Fire Girls (1910); Girl Scouts (1912); Pathfinders of America (1914). To these one can add, the Public Education Association of Philadelphia (1881), the Public Education Association of New York (1895), and Witmer's clinic (1896). The Juvenile Courts in Denver and in Chicago (1899), the visiting teacher movement (1906), and Healy's Juvenile Psychopathic Institute (1909) belong to the same period.

The turn of the century marked the beginning of the "Century of the Child" (Key, 1909; Kanner, 1962). The field of child study originated about this time in Europe as well as in the United States (Kessen, 1965). That professional clinical services for children were now

[1] Exceptions to this statement include institutions for the severe mental defective (Kanner, 1964), orphan asylums, and juvenile reformatories.

developing should occasion no surprise. A renewed and deepened concern for people, which encompassed all areas of health, education, and welfare, was part of the zeitgeist of this period.

Social Darwinism

In the United States, the concern with children grew out of the ferment accompanying great social and economic change. Increasing human misery forced attention to the human consequences of the industrialization and urbanization in the period following the Civil War when the railroad, mining, oil, steel, meat packing, and other industries flourished. The administrative and organizational genius of the early economic barons combined science, invention, and machinery in the development of techniques for large-scale production which both responded to, and encouraged the demands of a swiftly growing nation.

Industrial expansion was accompanied by rapid urbanization, and as we shall see, a mushrooming of social problems. In 1860, some 80 percent of the people lived in rural or farming environments. By 1920, nearly 60 percent lived in urban environments. In large proportion, those coming to the cities were immigrants drawn there by the voracious needs of an expanding industry for a labor force. After 1890, they were locked in by a closing frontier, and by the prohibitive costs of establishing a farm. Moreover, in the 1870's and 1880's farming was losing its attractiveness as an enterprise. Low farm prices, rising costs of transportation of farm products and manufactured goods, and financial policies sharply favoring creditors helped to depress the farmer and to accelerate the process of urbanization. In fact, at this time, the children of farmers started moving to the cities (Beard & Beard, 1927).

From one viewpoint, what happened to people in the period of progress following the Civil War was not important. Not only was government following a laissez-faire policy, but the intellectual spirit of the day supported the position of the man of affairs, as Eric Goldman (1956) showed so vividly. Liberty meant the right of a man to acquire and keep property without the interference of government. Competition was the correct means of distributing wealth. If the poor were poor, it was because they had too many children who ate up their incomes. Immigrant groups and Negroes were born to live in squalor and poverty for they lacked an inherited instinct for liberty. God gave man his abilities and any attempt to interfere with the use of those abilities was a violation of His will.

Herbert Spencer, the brilliant and facile English sociologist, came to America and was lionized because he formulated Social Darwinism, which held that society was an organism which evolved according to the laws of the survival of the fittest (Spencer, 1873). The businessman was adapted for survival, and social change, benefiting the poor and the halt, could result only in social disaster by interfering with "nature, red in fang and claw." As expounded by William Graham Sumner from his podium at Yale, such interference would weaken the race, threaten the economic system by placing an extreme burden on "the forgotten (middle-class) man," and fly in the face of American ideals of laissez-faire (Sumner, 1883; Davie, 1940; Hofstadter, 1955).

The concepts of Social Darwinism not only provided a philosophy for scholars and a rationale for the dominant classes, but also provided what Eric Goldman (1956) called "conservatism's steel chain of ideas"; there was actually no point in trying to change social institutions if people were born to live in a certain way.

A conservative philosophy holds the position that the problem resides within the person, and that corrective measures, if any, should change the person; the alternative viewpoint, that people are essentially good but are shaped by their environments, is generally characteristic of a liberal or reform philosophy.[2] As we shall try to show, the very form of professional practice in the mental health professions is shaped by whether the nation happens to be in a conservative or a reform period.

While social scientists or clinicians might protest at the idea that theories and methods of professional practice are shaped by political and social philosophy, it is a concept which deserves close attention. Pastore (1949) in a very worthwhile little monograph has shown an

[2] Staughton Lynd (personal communication) has suggested to us that two liberal or environmentalist positions need to be distinguished. One view holds that the human being is infinitely malleable in relation to changes in environment. Given that the goals of development are set, proponents of this view might be said to be "moral authoritarians." A second view holds that each man contains the "spark of the divine," an unknowable potential, which the best environment permits to emerge. This viewpoint necessarily demands tolerance of diversity, since it follows that each man should be helped to become the best he can be, given his potential.

important connection between a scientist's professional stand in the nature-nurture controversy and his public stand on political issues. Scientists who were political conservatives clearly favored the nature viewpoint. If one can discern such generalized attitudinal influences in public scientific positions, why should it not be possible that other aspects of scientific activity are also shaped in some degree by the spirit of the times?

the conditions for change

In that period of progress after the Civil War, not all was well with the system, and not all accepted their inferior positions passively. The depression of 1873 was followed by a great deal of disorder. On a political level, this era saw the development of the Populists, the Progressives, the Socialists, and the Anarchists. The labor movement began to come into its own, and its course over forty years was marked by strikes, violence, rioting, and the use of federal and state armed force to maintain order. There was widespread turmoil and fear of social conflict, or worse. Just as the threats and reality of urban riots provide the background for reforms in our day, so did violence and unrest set the climate for reform in that day.

The intellectuals of the day, moved by the wretched conditions of the poor, opposed the imperiousness of Social Darwinism and emphasized an environmental determinant of human behavior. Goldman (1956) and Hays (1957) both provide excellent views of the ferment in ideas which permitted social reformers not only to examine society, but to demand concrete reforms. Henry George (1873) decried the inevitable association of the increase in national wealth and poverty. The Muckrakers drew attention to abuses in industry. Lincoln Steffens (1904), and Jacob Riis (1902; 1917) focused on political corruption and life in the tenements. Religious leaders began to seek a Christian approach to the problems of the unfortunate (Hopkins, 1940; Abell, 1943). It was in this same period, between 1900 and 1917, that at least ten of the major philanthropic foundations were established, including the Russell Sage Foundation and the Commonwealth Fund, both so important in the development of social and clinical services for children.

The social justice movement, composed of lawyers, intellectuals, ministers, and upper-class women, sought change from state and federal legislatures which would enable the urban poor to rise above their circumstances (Hays, 1957). No small part of their work, and a good part of the work of the early settlement house workers, consisted in gathering data on the condition of women and children in the factories. Jane Addams (1910) for example describes in touching terms a debacle in which she attempted to use an ergograph to demonstrate that factory girls were indeed "dog-tired" after a long day.[3] To some extent, surveys and other types of empirical studies of the social environment developed because hard-headed legislators demanded proof that working conditions were indeed affecting women and children adversely. In fact, the science of sociology was seen as a means of promoting meaningful social reform (Hopkins, 1940; Abell, 1943).

There were severe problems of living in those days. The effects of the twin forces of industrialization and urbanization upon the individual, upon the family, and upon the sense of community were quite profound. In the case of the numerous immigrants, these effects were immeasurably compounded by the difficulties attendant upon changing entire ways of life (Handlin, 1951; 1959). Most of the immigrants were forced here by poor conditions in their own lands. They were largely unskilled, in terms of the needs of industrial society. One third were illiterate. They came from rural environments and were faced with the problem of adapting to the city as well as to the factory. Industrialization, with its tendency toward specialization of function, removed the worker from his household, subjected him to the external discipline of the factory, made him dependent upon the vagaries of the labor market for his existence, took away his sense of competence and his pride in his workmanship. A worker was no longer an individual in a community of individuals, with many diffused ties to others; his ties became role-specific, and his place in the group nebulous.

[3] Social scientists today look with pride on the fact that the 1954 Supreme Court recognized psychological studies in arriving at the decision that school segregation was inherently harmful. We generally forget that Louis Brandeis defended Oregon's ten-hour law for women before the Supreme Court in 1908 by making use of more than ninety reports, developed both through public and private auspices, which documented the fact that a ten-hour law was necessary to protect the health, safety, morals and general welfare of the people of Oregon. His arguments were accepted by the Supreme Court and helped to establish the precedent that the meaning given to the law should evolve in relation to social needs (Muller vs. Oregon, 1908; 208, US 412).

The urban stiuation made relationships more impersonal, utilitarian, and transitory. Primary group controls become less effective, and the social order was maintained by a variety of secondary institutional controls. The police, the social agencies, correctional agencies, investigating commissions, and the like became more important in the lives of people. These agencies, based upon explicit, impersonal rules, with powers of enforcement, took over bit by bit control functions which in former times were maintained by internalized folkways and mores governed by force of personal relationship (Wilensky & Lebeaux, 1965).

In place of the extended family, with the presence of many parents, the nuclear family became more important. Migration compounded family problems, for when men migrated first, as many did, sending for wives and children after saving up money for their passage, the families often suffered severe internal disruption. The smaller family intensified the ties among its members and, at the same time, the needs of the labor force drew more and more women out of the home, changing the role of women to some extent. With women being drawn into the factories and sweatshops to work long hours, under horrible conditions, often away from their children, the strain on the small family became even more acute. Divorce rates increased drastically, and, particularly in lower classes, families broken by divorce, desertion, or the premature death of one parent became more common. In simpler rural communities, with extended family ties, the broken family was not a social problem, for the community took care of its own. In the urban, industrial environment, specialized agencies became necessary.

Problems of youth were exacerbated. The place and value of children in the family had changed. As labor became more specialized, and as tasks in the home became more limited, children became less valuable economically and more dependent. This is not to say that children did not work. They did, both in factories and alongside their parents in the tenements. Some of the greatest abuses of this period were connected with child labor, an evil which was not really controlled until federal and state legislation in the 1930's and 1940's. The poverty of the period pulled children from the schools into the factories, but even the factories required minimally educated workers and citizens.

The schools, geared to the educational needs of the wealthier, native American groups, proved to have a curriculum and teaching methods irrelevant to the needs of immigrants who were going to enter the factories, and then, as now, the school system changed slowly and with difficulty. Reformers, intellectuals, and scientists recognized that irrelevant and inadequate school programs were forcing children out of school, contributing to delinquency, and creating human waste. Jane Addams (1910) tells us she became a member of the Chicago School Board precisely because she hoped to be able to influence school programs to change, thus reducing a cause of delinquency.

In the days of immigration children assimilated much faster than their parents, making for intergenerational conflict and a reduction in the authority and influence of the older generation. Delinquency, school problems, and the like tended to occur with greatest frequency in the first generation of immigrant children born on American soil.

social problems among the Jews

From about 1890 on, eastern European Jews, fleeing pogroms, restrictive legislation, and economic recession in their homelands, had come to the United States in large numbers. They came to the cities at the same time as the Italians and other south and central European peoples. These groups displaced the northern Europeans from the oldest and poorest sections of the cities.

Many people believe that in the "good old days," people were poor, but because they had close knit families, because they worked hard, and because they sacrificed for their children to go to schools, they pulled themselves up by their bootstraps. Today, some make invidious comparisons between the earlier immigrants and today's Negro and Puerto Rican urban poor. In general, the stereotyped view is only partially correct, for what it denies is the degree to which there were social problems among all of these immigrant groups, even the Jews, who are often offered as the outstanding example of successful immigrant adaptation (Glazer & Moynihan, 1963).

In the course of the present research we encountered a great deal which suggested that a variety of social problems, not dissimilar to those of the present day, were endemic among all immigrant groups, including the Jews. The evidence we uncovered was startling to us, and startling to those friends and colleagues to whom we related it.

While none were experts in this particular period of history, their surprise, in confirmation of our own, made us feel that many of our readers would also find the evidence engrossing and thought provoking.

We feel it is worthwhile to present some of the data as background for understanding why there was a need for professional helping services. What follows will center on the Jews as a group because we believe the revelation that there were severe problems will bring home the point that any group, white or black, Jew or Gentile, exposed to the conditions of severe urban poverty will develop a similar set of social problems. We feel this evidence not only enlightens us concerning the reasons for the development of the many helping services, but it also helps to put present-day inner-city problems in better perspective.

family disorganization

Jacob Riis (1917), the reformer concerned with New York City's urban problems, described New York's all Jewish Tenth Ward, the Lower East Side, as having the greatest population density known in any country, and that population was housed in overpriced, overcrowded tenements. He said that to the health officers of the city it was known as the "typhus ward," and to the official body which dealt with suicides as the "suicide ward." It was known "among the police as the 'crooked ward' on account of the number of 'crooks', petty thieves and their allies, the 'fences', receivers of stolen goods who find the dense crowds congenial." Confirmation of the presence of many severe social problems among the Jews may be found in Goren (1966).

Jewish family life in the miserably crowded and filthy cities was not as close or as problem-free as we have been taught to believe. "It is doubtful that there were specific relief needs peculiar to the Jewish population in the United States, aside from religious and cultural considerations, despite recurrent concern that this might be the case. *Thus, desertion in the early 1900's was considered to be a 'Jewish problem' and a major cause of dependency in Jewish families. However, subsequent investigations proved that desertion was at least as common, if not more so among non-Jewish families"* (Italics ours) (Stein, 1958, p. 201).

An example of the family disorganization present is found in a description of a child treated in Witmer's clinic in Philadelphia. The child was an eight-year-old girl, of Russian-Jewish parentage, brought to the clinic because she had spent two years in first grade with no progress. She was brought not by her parents, but by a visiting nurse. She was described as one of seven children, poorly nourished, dull, sullen, and unwilling or unable to answer simple questions. Her home was described as follows:

> The living room has one window, contains a table, a few chairs, a stove and lounge, no carpet, dirty clothes piled in one corner, many flies and a barking dog. The table is covered with a piece of black oil cloth on which there is usually to be found pieces of brown bread and glasses of tea. . . . The family never sits down to the table; no meals are prepared. . . . Bread is always on the table and the children take it up when they feel like eating. . . . One hydrant at the entrance suffices for the different families; there is underground drainage, but an offensive odor comes from the water closets (Witmer, 1907, p. 143).

Anyone with any experience in our urban slums of today will recognize the child and her family.

Confirmation of problems in family stability comes indirectly from an analysis of themes which were popular on the Yiddish stage in those days. Hutchins Hapgood (1967), in a sympathetic study of the Jewish quarter, now considered a classic, describes the Yiddish theatre's melodramatic portrayals of the living problems of the Jewish poor in the new world. The tremendously popular plays abounded in the suicides of fallen women, illicit sexual relationships between wives or daughters and the ubiquitous boarder, and marital difficulties stemming from changes in life-style wrought by the new environment. A not infrequent villain was the cruel husband.

Unwed mothers were by no means rare. The Kimpetoran Society, formed to alleviate distressing conditions among indigent Jewish mothers on New York's Lower East Side, listed many husbandless young mothers among the recipients of "a scuttle of coal, a clean bed-sheet, a few diapers, and $5" (Lukas, 1967).

Some of the more important problems arose when the first generation began to break away from old customs and from the authority of its parents. Many stories and plays described the ensuing heartbreak. Lincoln Steffens (1931) describes, as more than occasional, fights in ghetto homes between fathers who attempted to control their children by physical punishment, and young toughs who did not hesitate to strike back. The fights were severe enough to bring the police.

delinquency

Delinquency was apparently a common problem in that area, and the delinquency was by no means always of a minor nature.

"The young people of Jewtown are inordinately fond of dancing,[4] and after their hard day's work will flock to these 'dancing schools' for a night's recreation . . . . it happens that a school adjourns in a body to make a general raid on the rival establishment across the street, without the ceremony of paying the admission fee. Then the dance breaks up in a general fight, in which likely enough someone is badly hurt. The police come in, as usual, and ring down the curtain" (Riis, 1917, p. 110).

The problem was not restricted to New York's Lower East Side. At least 7 percent of Healy's (1915) 1,000 delinquents in Chicago were of Russian-Jewish parentage, and judging from the listing of other Eastern European birthplaces of his group, as many as 15 or 20 percent of the youth may have been Jewish. About 70 percent of all delinquents had foreign-born parents while the native-born white population of Chicago produced only 14.5 percent of all delinquents. Healy deliberately avoids giving a breakdown by religious grouping, saying it would do no good. He also points out that Jews were seen in unusual numbers in his clinic because of the efforts of Jewish fraternal and social agencies to look after their own delinquents. At the very least, it must be said that Jewish delinquents were not rare in Chicago around 1910.

In Philadelphia, it was estimated that 20 percent of all delinquents coming before the Juvenile Court were Jews. The same source indicates that the Juvenile Court in Philadelphia specifically selected a Yiddish-speaking probation worker to help them cope with the problems

[4] Do you think they all had rhythm?

(International Prison Commission, 1904). In Denver, the reports of the Juvenile Court for the years 1908 to 1910 list figures by religious group. Between 16 and 20 percent of all children who came before the Juvenile Court were Jews (Denver and Arapahoe County Juvenile Court Report, 1908–1909; 1909–1910). Several of the boys mentioned in one of Judge Lindsey's books had Jewish names, while it is specifically stated that half of one of the gangs which worked with Lindsey was composed of Jewish children. Moreover, some of Lindsey's strongest support as a political independent came from the families of Russian Jewish boys whom he had befriended (Lindsey & O'Higgins, 1910). An undated pamphlet from the Juvenile Court in Denver, describing the State Industrial School at Golden, states that teachers from Denver gave religious instruction to Jewish boys on Sunday afternoons.

Further evidence of delinquent and criminal activity among the Jews on the Lower East Side may be found in Gold's novel, *Jews Without Money* (Gold, 1930), while Coulter (1913), clerk of the Juvenile Court, and founder of the Big Brother movement in New York, implies, but does not state, that faginism (teaching young children to steal) and pickpocketing were largely Jewish enterprises on the Lower East Side. Riis (1902) states that the fighting gangs among the Irish were matched by the thieving gangs among the Jews. As late as 1930, fully 20 percent of the children brought to the attention of the Juvenile Court in New York City were Jewish. While it is true that more than a third of the Jewish offenses in 1930 were for peddling or begging without a license, a sizeable proportion were for other, more anti-social acts. By 1952, Jewish children seen in the New York City courts had dropped to 3 percent, a tenth of the rate expected if Jewish children were to appear in Juvenile Court in proportion to their numbers (Robison, 1958).

The available evidence suggests then that delinquency of all kinds was by no means uncommon among the Jews who came to the cities in the pre-World War I days. Since there was a fairly high rate of delinquency among the Jews in cities as widespread as New York, Philadelphia, Chicago, and Denver, one can say that urban conditions poverty, crowding, and unfamiliarity with the ways of the city produced common effects. Our assumption is that crime and delinquency were probably more prevalent among other immigrant groups in the cities, and the literature of the time presents ample evidence of rowdyism, thieving, fighting, gangsterism, attacks on police by crowds in the streets, and the myriad other anti-social disorders among almost every one of the immigrant groups.

prostitution

Evidence of delinquency occasions surprise, but evidence of the extent of involvement of Jews in prostitution in that day is still more surprising. We began looking into the evidence on prostitution when we noted mention of the openness and prevalence of prostitution among the Jews in the works of Jane Addams (1910), Lincoln Steffens (1931), and Michael Gold (1930). Lincoln Steffens and Gold describe nearly identical scenes in which children, through the windows of their own tenements, view prostitutes entertaining their customers. The Lower East Side had a long standing reputation as a red-light district, a reputation well confirmed in the story about the first visitor to the College Settlement, which was located in a district settled largely by Russian and Polish Jews. That visitor was a policeman who unwittingly described the neighborhood and his relationship with it by asking for a bribe not to interfere with the business activities of the seven young women (Davis, 1959). Lillian Wald (1915), most famous of the visiting nurses, delicately refers to the few blocks of the red-light district near her Henry Street Settlement in New York which, for years, she would not enter out of a sense of shame.

Prostitution was widespread in the country, and Jews were heavily involved, both as prostitutes and as procurers. Maude Emma Miner, the Secretary of the New York Probation and Protective Association, cites a number of case histories of prostitutes in New York (Miner, 1916). The names she gives them, perhaps a quarter of the cases according to our count, are Rose Schafer, Rachel Goldberg, Sophie Bergman, Yetta Rosen, Bertha Levy, and Jennie Rosenberg. When a Jewish name is mentioned, there is no statement to attest that the Jewish prostitute was rare. On the contrary, Miner writes, with great sympathy: "It is a comparatively new phenomenon in the life of the

Hebrew people to have any of its daughters in prostitution. The moral standards of Jewish women have been high. Less than a generation ago it was rare in New York City for a Jewish girl to be living a life of prostitution. Now many are entering the life" (Miner, 1916, p. 35).

The presence of Jewish prostitutes is matched by the extent to which Jews were involved in the organization of prostitution. Miner reports data from the Report of the U.S. Immigration Commission on the Importation and Harboring of Women for Immoral Purposes (Senate Document, No. 196, 1909, p. 23). In a group of 218 procurers, 65 percent were Russian or Italian, and in that day there were few Russian immigrants other than Jews. The report goes on to state that "there were two organizations of importance, one French, the other Jewish"; and further, "the activity of Jewish procurers in seducing young girls and turning them into prostitution was much greater than the French, whereas the French were more willing to import women who were already familiar with the life."

In discussing prosecutions of procurers, Miner states that Morris and Lena Cohen boasted of having the largest clearing house for women in New York City; another procurer named Samuel Rubin was given a long-term sentence for that crime. Confirmation for the presence of Jews in prostitution is found in the Report of the Moral Survey Committee of Syracuse, New York (1913). The following is an excerpt from the investigator's report: "Visited Madame X-9's parlor house, X-10. Met there a girl I know. She introduced me to the madam as one of the boys. I stated my errand to Syracuse, to open a house if possible, as New York is now so 'tight'. She discouraged me by informing me that 'they' will not stand for Jews, that the minute a Jew opens up, they get to citizen X-11 who gets to official X-12 and has them driven from the town. I explained to her that my woman is a Gentile and that I wouldn't mix in."

The fact that the undercover investigator was Jewish and openly identified himself as such to the madam speaks for itself. We have found similar references to Jewish cadets (a term for pimp) and Jewish prostitutes in reports from Hartford, Connecticut (Hartford Vice Commission, 1913), and in a pamphlet entitled "Facts for Mothers and Fathers" issued in New York about this same time. Many of the other reports of vice commissions from cities throughout the country contain similar data on prostitution, but one cannot discern the ethnic backgrounds of the people involved because individuals are identified by case number only. However indication of birthplace of the individual or of the parents in Eastern European countries is not infrequent, and a substantial proportion of these may have been Jews.

A Jewish source, a report of the International Society for the Rescue of Jewish Women and Children (1927), documents the problem of white slavery among the Jews. They do not provide any figures, and the participants (including Bertha Pappenheim, who was probably Freud and Breuer's Anna O. [Oberndorf, 1953] and at this time a well-functioning social worker), differ among themselves about the extent of the problem in the post-World War I era. However, they are clear in indicating there was indeed a sizeable problem in the pre-war period. This source describes in great detail, and in a form sufficiently melodramatic to rival the best of the productions of the Yiddish stage, the tragedy of young women who were forced into the life. Immigration had resulted in a shortage of young men in the *shtetlach* (villages). Sharp operators would come to the villages and say they had husbands in the new world, for many were introduced into prostitution by cadets the proxy ceremony, the girls would be loaded aboard ships and taken to Hong Kong, to South America, and to the United States where they would be delivered to brothels and held in literal slavery. The rescue society described raids on ships in which the group would forcibly release women from the clutches of their captors.

Apparently it was not easy for a young woman to find a husband in the new world, for many were introduced into prostitution by cadets who falsely promised to marry the girls, or who took advantage of the girls' naivete by entering into fraudulent marriages with them. In many instances, however, the motivation to enter prostitution was a desire to escape the hard, drab life of sweatshops and tenements, and to satisfy a yearning for the fineries that the uptown shops provided for wealthy uptown women. The problem may have been more common among the first American-born generation than among its immigrant sisters, just as delinquency may have been in some part a function of the intergenerational gap. The existence of the problem in the early 1900's, in the "good old days," may give us a somewhat more sympathetic understanding of ghetto youth of today who see hustling and prostitution as their way of adapting to and conquering the hard life of the city.

the public schools

It has been generally accepted that the Eastern European Jews did exceptionally well in the public schools. Lillian Wald (1915) is one among many who described how the Jewish parent urged education upon his child, willingly making great sacrifices to support his education. Jacob Riis (1917) also mentions that the eager Jewish students quickly became top scholars taking all of the prizes in schools they attended. Lincoln Steffens (1931), Hutchins Hapgood (1967), and others described the vigorous intellectual life among the young adults in the Jewish ghetto. While the general picture is undoubtedly true, there is another side of the educational picture which has been neglected. When we see the nature of the educational problem among the educationally oriented immigrant Jews, we can understand that the problem was considerably worse among other groups. The schools themselves contributed heavily to the problem of education.

In the generation preceding the Civil War, the fight for free public schools and universal education had been largely won, but placing the schools under the aegis of the politician did nothing to help promote rapid change when change became necessary. The normal schools for teacher training made their appearance before the Civil War and education quickly fell victim to professionalization, bureaucratization, and a variety of corrupt political influences. By the 1870's the city schools began to feel the burden of a school population rapidly increasing as a result of immigration, urbanization, and the new compulsory attendance laws. The schools responded by developing rigid systems for grade level, pupil promotion, and supervision of instruction, as well as all the other institutional trappings so essential to processing masses of people and so antithetical to individual needs.

In these and subsequent years, the immigrants along with migrants from the farms continued to flood the badly lighted, poorly heated, unsanitary schools. Class sizes in excess of sixty were all too common. By 1909, more than 57 percent of the children in the 37 largest school districts in the United States were of foreign-born parentage. In New York and in Chicago, at least two-thirds of the children were of foreign-born parentage (Cremin, 1964).

One of the critical factors in the problems faced by schools was the compulsory school attendance laws. The fight for universal, free, tax-supported public schools had been more or less won earlier, but until 1852, no state required attendance at school. Between 1870 and 1890, the bulk of compulsory school attendance laws were passed, and by 1912, every state in the union had such a law. These laws were passed for a variety of motives. Labor unions were in favor of them as a means of curbing child labor, and frequently compulsory school attendance laws were passed in tandem with child labor laws. The laws were favored by humanitarian reformers not only because they struck at child labor, but because they held promise of creating a literate populace, an indispensable prerequisite for a democratic society.

As with many good ideas, the implementation left much to be desired. These laws, forcing an overwhelming population on the schools, indirectly provided the single most important force in the development of clinical services for children, and eventually for change in school programs. The laws were passed, and the problems thereby created for the schools were immediate and immense.[5] Over the years 1890–1920, the nation's population increased by 68 percent, the public school population increased by 70 percent, and average daily attendance increased almost 100 percent, reflecting enforcement of the attendance laws.

More children were coming into school and more children were retained in school to an older age, but the school was in no way prepared for the onslaught. We can do no better than quote from Monroe (1911) who wrote about the status of compulsory school attendance laws before the 1890's as follows.

> From the start it has been found that the satisfactory execution of attendance laws requires special adjustments within the schools. Children forced to come to school against their will, or with little interest in school cannot be classified with children who attend regularly. . . . unless special schools are provided. The school authorities them-

[5] Then as now, solutions to problems are written into the laws, without adequate consideration for dealing with other consequences. Laws are written by politicians, not by social scientists, who sometimes find the laws contribute to mental health problems. In many states, youth are permitted by law to leave school at age 16. However, other laws, child labor and workmen's compensation, effectively bar such youth from many industrial employment opportunities. The laws thus contribute to the conditions which promote adolescent delinquency.

selves will hardly cooperate in enforcing the law if such is not the case. New York State passed its first compulsory law in 1874. After fourteen years' trial, it was found that the law had not modified school attendance, had not secured the cooperation of school principals and was most substantially a dead letter. The machinery for its execution was inadequate, but at bottom it was a question of lack of accommodation for the difficult pupil (p. 294).

It was a similar circumstance in France which led to the development of the intelligence test. France had passed a compulsory public education act in 1882, with provision for its enforcement. By 1904, the French Ministry of Public Instruction knew it had a problem on its hands. Children were coming to school and not adapting to the school as it existed. Alfred Binet and Theodore Simon were commissioned to devise methods for selecting children who could not adapt to the regular curriculum and who thereby reduced the efficiency of teachers and other children. The intelligence test was developed as part of the planning for the introduction of special classes into the public schools (Peterson, 1926). The social class bias in intelligence tests and the profound consequences for the definition of intelligence have been developed by Eels et al. (1951).

By the 1890's, when Southern and Eastern Europeans began to arrive by the hundreds of thousands, the schools were faced with further problems. The newcomers could not cope with the school's rigid curriculum, and one result was the retention of large numbers of pupils. When the term retardation was used originally it did not necessarily mean retardation in terms of mental and physical growth. It meant that students were overage for their grade. The extent of the problem in the urban schools of the time is revealed in a number of reports. In the schools of Camden, New Jersey, in 1905–1906, fully 26 percent of the pupils were two or more years behind according to the pioneering investigation reported by Superintendent of Schools Bryant (1906). Cornman (1906) reported figures for a variety of grades and found that in New York 30 percent were retarded, in Boston, 22 percent, in Philadelphia 37 percent, and in Kansas City, almost 50 percent. The differences between cities reflect administrative regulation as much as differences in the kinds of people who settled in the cities.[6] Heilman (1906) cites similar figures by way of making a case for the need for special classes in the public schools.

Successive issues of Witmer's *Psychological Clinic* reflect the deep consideration given to school retardation. Bryant attributed the problem to the "serious efforts to enforce provisions of compulsory education enactments [which] have led to the presence of large numbers of children who are unable to make steady progress in the school."[7]

Although there were a few sporadic efforts in the United States to open special classes in the 1870's, the first special classes did not begin until 1896. By 1905, the idea of special classes, classes originally begun as disciplinary units, and not to take care of intellectual needs, had taken hold. Most of the larger cities had these, but in insufficient numbers to meet the need. But then as now, the public at large had so little understanding of the problems the school faced that the first such special class was greeted by an article in the local paper calling it the "Fool Class" (Kanner, 1964).

Lightner Witmer, whom we shall discuss in the next chapter, was one of the leaders in developing the special class. He helped the Philadelphia school system organize special classes, and with others (Van Sickle, Witmer, & Ayres, 1911), wrote an important monograph on special classes. He promoted the special class concept through his journal, *The Psychological Clinic,* seeing the special class as a means of treating children with special educational needs. Witmer did not intend to remove problems from the regular school. On the contrary, *he intended to use special classes as a means of providing for individual differences within the framework of the regular public school.* An editorial in *The Psychological Clinic* (1908) introducing two articles on special classes clearly reveals his view that the introduction of special classes into the school system was part of the reform of the school system in relation to the failure of the school to provide adequate education for all children.[8]

---

[6] In later years the problem was solved by the simple expedient of promoting almost everyone, by administrative fiat.

[7] The efforts of enforcement in part represent the work and interest of reformers of the social justice movement. Jane Addams (1925), for example, describes how one of her settlement workers undertook an intensive study of pupil attendance in Chicago schools. Abbott and Breckinridge (1917), two former Hull House workers, also reported on attendance in the schools in Chicago.

[8] The editorial also makes explicit Witmer's conception of the classroom teacher as an applied psychologist and the special classroom as the clinical psychologist's laboratory.

The nature of these classes and the problems the immigrant children presented to the public schools is admirably depicted in a report written by Helena T. Devereux, one of the very early special class teachers. She later went on to found and develop the Devereux Schools, presently the largest private residential treatment center for retarded and emotionally disturbed children. Her report. quoted almost in full, with some extraneous detail omitted, offers a view of the classroom from the vantage point of the teacher.

On January 15, 1908, a class for exceptional children was formed in a large school in the foreign slum district of Philadelphia. . . . These children were reported not only as being stupid, but "queer." It is hard to define exactly what was meant by this term but it did mean that the child to whom it was applied was singled out from the other children. Other children not placed in the class were dull and slow but still normal, while each of these children seemed to have a personality differing from the normal child and also from the purely incorrigible type.

From January, 1908 to February, 1909, forty-three children have attended the class, some for one month and some for the year, some for both sessions and some for only one. Among these children thirty-four were of Russian Hebrew extraction and four of Italian. Of the twenty-six who first formed the class, six were respectably cared for. The others were much neglected, and as they lacked even the pride of the ordinary child, they were, indeed a forlorn looking little company, insufficiently fed and poorly clothed. They ranged in ages from eight to fifteen years, being from two to five years retarded as compared with the average child. . . .

Before the class was started the idea was that the manual work (woodwork, basketry, paper, sloyd, and sewing) might be a means of awakening the child and might form a "peg" on which to hang the real mental training. My only idea was to immediately teach the child the rudiment of school work and so return it to the regular grade when it was sufficiently advanced. When I had been with the class for one week I abandoned my scheme of memory and sense perception, training the intellect only as a side issue, and I determined to base all my work on the development of the emotions. The great need of those children as I read it then was to make them less like little animals— to instill humanity into them. I could understand then wherein these children were queer. They were subnormal or rather freakish in disposition and temperament. They were selfwilled, passionate, malicious, and all their shortcomings were very glaring, largely because they had not the sense of their fellows to see when it was expedient to be "good." With each child I picked out the moral defect or defects which were most emphasized such as selfishness, untruthfulness, stubbornness and temper, and determined to overcome them. I tried to make them see in every way what was the right thing to do, and not only to make them do it but to make them want to do it. I cared less that they should learn to write their names or finish an article in woodwork beautifully than that they should learn truthfulness, obedience and promptness, and truly they learned to watch, to listen, and to do. The bearing that this phase of the work, the training of the emotions, had upon the results cannot be overestimated. It laid the foundation for the other training —the mental side. I certainly agree with the educators who say that when once the real personality of the backward child is revealed it is more childlike in its trust, kindliness and simplicity than the normal child. When once they recognized that the teacher was their friend their attitude towards school life gradually changed. When definite instruction for the purpose of advancing them in their school work was given, the children were earnest little workers who wanted to learn. Their previous training had increased their power of attention so that the teaching was comparatively easy. I found each child had some serious defect, such as the inability to do arithmetic, written language, or reading. Even now when they are returned to the grade, some still have a persistent defect but it does not mar their entire standing. . . .

This class has in one year been a blessing to thirty-three [sic] children, children who, though never doomed by nature to spend their lives in an institution, would surely have drifted to one, which in some cases might easily have been a prison, had not some interest been taken in them. This class was begun amid many difficulties, there being no public funds provided for the necessary materials. Then too, the work was marred by my inexperience. The success of the class, especially as far as the regeneration of the boys is concerned, has been achieved largely through the wood-work which was the basis of manual, emotional and mental training, and that was made possible by the generosity of a Philadelphia merchant. May my last word be a plea for more classes in our city, properly equipped, where the three-fold motto shall be interest, persistency and encouragement to aid in making useful men and women out of "the least of God's little ones" (Devereux, 1909, pp. 45–48).

educational problems among the Jews

The reader might already have noted that Helena Devereux (1909) reported that 34 of 43 children in her special class in Philadelphia were Russian-Jewish in origin. In an earlier article, Heilman (1906), in presenting the need for special classes in the Philadelphia schools, described 20 cases of retarded children in need of special schooling. Of these 20 children, no fewer than 12 were of Russian-Jewish origin,[9] while four were Italian. The remainder were Irish, Swedish, German, and native born.

[9] While we will present evidence that many Jewish children were not successful in the public schools, there is no evidence, nor should anyone draw the implication that retardation was specifically a Jewish problem. We do know that by and large Jewish children did well in the schools. We don't know how many of the immigrant and first generation children did poorly in the schools. We suspect the numbers may have been sizable, but we do not know and have not seen that the problem was studied along religious or ethnic lines.

The visiting teacher, forerunner of the school social worker, began work in the urban slums. In New York, in Boston, and in Hartford, Connecticut, some of the first visiting teachers were placed in school districts from 81 to 96 percent Jewish. The problems these visiting teachers handled included deficient scholarship, truancy, incorrigibility, adverse home conditions, and neglect. There is no evidence to indicate the problems were any more frequent among Jews than among other groups, but clearly the problems were of sufficient frequency to warrant placing some of the visiting teachers in schools in predominantly Jewish neighborhoods (National Association of Visiting Teachers, 1921). Another indication of the problems in education may be found in the fact that in the early 1900's a type of school which would now be called a "600" school was established on the predominantly Jewish Lower East Side.

In general, the poor and dirty slum-dwelling Jews were not always received with open arms by the public schools. Jacob Riis pointed out that some of the children of "Jewtown" went to religious schools. "But the majority of the children seek the public schools, where they are received with some misgivings on the part of teachers, who find it necessary to inculcate lessons of cleanliness in the worst cases by practical demonstration with washbowl and soap" (Riis, 1917, p. 113).

We are wont to speak now of the cultural difference between the middle-class teacher and the lower-class child. The problem was no different around the turn of the century. The following passage is from *Jews Without Money*, a novel written by Michael Gold, who was born on the Lower East Side in 1894. Although the novel was popular in the 1930's and is considered one of the protest pieces of the time, it is largely autobiographical, and one can safely assume Gold is depicting his own public school experience in the early 1900's.

> I first admired Nigger[10] in school, when I was new there. He banged the teacher on the nose.
>
> School is a jail for children. One's crime is youth and the jailers punish one for it. I hated school at first; I missed the street. It made me nervous to sit stiffly in a room while New York blazed with autumn.
>
> I was always in hot water. The fat old maid teacher (weight about 250 pounds), with a sniffle, and eyeglasses, and the waddle of a ruptured person was my enemy.

[10] Nigger was not a Negro, but a white Jew; Nigger was his nickname.

She was shocked by the dirty word, I, a six-year-old villain, once used. She washed my mouth with yellow lye soap. I submitted. She stood me in the corner for the day to serve as an example of anarchy to a class of fifty scared kids.

Soap eating is nasty. But my parents objected because soap is made of Christian fat, is not kosher. I was being forced into pork-eating, a crime against the Mosaic law. They complained to the principal.

O irritable, starched old maid teacher, O stupid proper, unimaginative despot, O cow with no milk or calf or bull, it was torture to you, Ku Kluxer before your time, to teach in a Jewish neighborhood.

I knew no English when handed to you. I was a little savage and lover of the street. I used no toothbrush. I slept in my underwear, I was lousy, maybe. To sit on a bench made me restless, my body hated coffins. But Teacher! O Teacher for little slaves, O ruptured American virgin of fifty-five, you should not have called me "LITTLE KIKE!"

Nigger banged you on the nose for that. I should have been as brave. It was Justice (Gold, 1930, pp. 22–23).

some speculations

It may be worth speculating why the evidence of social problems, of Jewish delinquency, family instability, of involvement in prostitution, and of school problems has been forgotten. There was, of course, much to be proud of in the Jewish group. There *were* very many self-sacrificing mothers and fathers. There *were* very many good students. The second generation *did* have less difficulty than the immigrant or the first generation, and by the third, anti-social problems had almost disappeared.

In addition, popular writers who were not Jewish, such as Hapgood, Steffens, and even Jacob Riis (he spoke of the stubborn people of "Jewtown" who refused to recognize Christ) were very much attracted to the Jewish intellectual group, for there *was* a vigorous artistic and intellectual life in the ghetto. These writers made Jewish friends and came to understand the culture in its many dimensions. Moreover, these writers were liberal reformers, eager to bring about social change in the corrupt municipalities of the time. While immigration was largely unchecked until after the First World War, there were many who saw the immigrants as a distinct threat to the well-being of American society. Many of the liberal writers of the day felt compelled to point out the immigrant contribution to the American economy and to American culture by way of defending the presence of the immigrants, and by way of supporting efforts at reform. Taking account of open anti-semitism, reform-oriented writers may have felt it advisable and necessary to minimize reports of Jewish anti-social behavior. Since many of the social scientists of that time were also reformers, the problem of Jewish involvement in anti-social phenomenon may not have been studied. Healy (1915), for example, tells us that he deliberately suppressed data showing the rate at which the different religious groups produced delinquents. Jews may also have received favorable attention because of the sobriety of the group. The literature emphasizes there were no Jewish alcoholics, and this in a time when prohibition was a favorite cause among reformers.

The adaptation of the Jews in America is all the more remarkable, considering the extent to which there were social problems among them. The factors contributing to the sharp reduction in social problems in a relatively few years deserve close attention for the lesson the earlier time may hold for today. The contribution of the Jewish welfare and social agencies and the tradition of self-help in the Jewish community is worthy of detailed study in light of contemporary understanding of social process. *But above all, we should recognize that miserable social conditions produced a high incidence of anti-social behavior, even among the Jews. That anti-social behavior died down in direct proportion to the prosperity of the country and the prosperity of the Jewish group is a lesson worth underscoring.*

summary

Our historical and social survey of the period has shown that the turn of the century was a strongly reform period, that there was considerable social unrest at the time, and that various social institutions were plagued with a host of troubles stemming from immigration, industrialization, urbanization, and poverty. As part of the general reform movement, there was concern about the way in which men lived; man himself necessarily had become a subject of intellectual interest. It was in this context that reformers and intellectuals took an interest in the schools, in children, and in their welfare. In the next chapters we shall describe the helping facilities, Witmer's clinic, the settlement houses, the Juvenile Court, the visiting teacher, and Healy's Juvenile Psychopathic Institute, all of which grew directly out of this context of social unrest and reform.

4

the first psychological clinic— Lightner Witmer, 1896

To add to the troubles of the public school system, the schools, then as now, received attention from a vast variety of educational "experts." The basic reason is not hard to find. John Dewey (1897) expressed the viewpoint of intellectuals and reformers when he said, "I believe that education is the fundamental method of social progress and reform." Clearly anyone who wanted society to be different saw that the schools were the first point of attack. Cremin (1964) has documented the history of the progressive education movement and has shown the variety of changes wrought through the years by Dewey, his followers, and others. The sterile formal methodology, the irrelevance of the curriculum to the real world, the lack of manual training, and corrupt political influences were variously attacked by muckrakers and other intellectuals. The vulnerability of the schools caused by their myriad problems was an important factor in obtaining some degree of curricular change.

The attention the intellectuals, particularly those in the university community, gave to education is worth recording, because it provides some significant background for Witmer's interest in the public schools and his decision to establish an applied service. Dewey had gone to the University of Chicago in 1894 to head the departments of philosophy, psychology, and pedagogy. The University of Chicago at that time was the heartland of reform Darwinism. In 1896, the chairman of its sociology department, Albion Small, had addressed the National Education Association and in resounding terms insisted the school was the prime medium for social change. Dewey, at that time a respected philosopher and psychologist, was on Jane Addams' board and contributed to some degree to the development of the educational program at Hull House.

Earlier, G. Stanley Hall had given lectures to teachers on educational problems, and when he came to Clark, he formed a department of pedagogy there. In 1891 he began the *Pedagogical Seminary*, a journal devoted to the new scientific approach to education (Hall, 1923). By 1895 courses were offered in the new pedagogy in at least five major universities. In 1899, Teachers College became part of Columbia University and E. L. Thorndike began to develop educational psychology as a respectable field of study (Boring, 1957).

Among other American intellectuals who took an interest in the public schools was William James. In 1892, he delivered a series of lectures to the public school teachers of Cambridge entitled "Talks to Teachers." These popular lectures were delivered by James throughout the country and finally appeared in book form in 1899 (James, 1899). In these lectures, James tried to show what the New Psychology had to say about the learning and the teaching process.

The topic of education was in the air, for the *Psychological Review* of 1897 records a controversy between Hugo Munsterberg, the founder of applied psychology, and James McKeen Cattell, who was Witmer's predecessor as Director of the Psychological Laboratories at the University of Pennsylvania. It would not be difficult to reproduce the terms of the argument today in academic circles. Munsterberg argued with force and conviction that the New Psychology, experimental laboratory psychology, had nothing whatever to say to the public school teacher, because it was irrelevant. Cattell, defending the experimental method, said the findings of psychology were solidly established in laboratory research, and that eventually the scientific soundness of experimental psychology would enable it to make its contribution. In the meantime Cattell was satisfied that the New Psychology was scientific.

Given the problems the schools were experiencing and the interest of eminent psychologists, philosophers, and sociologists in the public school system, it is not surprising that when Lightner Witmer developed the first psychological clinic in the United States, if not the world, at the University of Pennsylvania in 1896, that clinic was focused on educational issues.

Witmer (1915) himself tells how his clinic was a product of broader social forces. In a public lecture given in 1913, Witmer discussed the history of services for the exceptional child, giving recognition to the work of Pereire, Seguin, Pinel, Itard, and the other pioneers in work with the mentally retarded. He referred to this earlier work as the first movement. He goes on to say:

> The second movement for the study and educational treatment of exceptional children was inspired, or at least made possible by the development of modern science, especially psychology and hygiene. It began about the year 1890 in this country, and was the result of the introduction of school medical inspection, the enforcement of compulsory education, the failure of society to provide for the care of the blind, deaf, feebleminded and delinquent children, the development of a type of applied psychology called clinical psychology, and lastly the increased efficiency of public school administration, which led to the discovery that millions of children in the United States were not obtaining the elementary education which they were supposed to be getting and which a democracy insists is necessary for self governing citizenship.
>
> The earlier movement for the training of exceptional children was not conceived as part of the problem of general education. It was in part a scientific movement and in part a humanitarian movement. To some extent also it was a blind effort of society at self preservation by removing from society (temporarily at least) certain unfit elements. The later movement for the educational treatment of exceptional children is a part of the public school problem. It represents a conscious effort to introduce scientific procedure into common school practice. It has had and will

have far reaching consequences not only upon educational practice with respect to all children but also upon the development of the sciences of psychology and hygiene. It led directly to the founding of psychological clinics at the University of Pennsylvania and other institutions of learning, and to the establishment of similar clinics in connection with the public school system of many cities. . . .

I have taken part in this movement for the more scientific treatment of exceptional children from its inception in this country, and from the beginning I have been inspired by the belief that the study and training of the exceptional child constituted the most favorable point of approach for a psychology applied to educational practice (Witmer, 1915, pp. 535–537).

Although Lightner Witmer was very much the academician and the experimental scientist, in keeping with the spirit of the times Witmer turned his attention toward practical problems, aligning himself with Thomas Huxley in a belief in the continuity of pure and applied science (Witmer, 1906). The lecture quoted above was written nearly twenty years after the beginning of the first clinic, but his earliest writings expressed the same ideas. In the first written description of the clinic, a paper read at a meeting of the American Psychological Association in 1896, Witmer (1897) indicated his interest in working out a relationship between the psychology department and the public schools. In the second volume of his journal, *The Psychological Clinic,* Witmer openly stated in an editorial that both the clinic and the journal were "propagandistic in spirit." He stated that it was his purpose to urge upon the school the realization of its possibilities as a social force, as an institution essential for "the development of the individual and the progress of the race" (Witmer, 1908).

His clinic began in the spring of 1896 as part of the psychology department of the University of Pennsylvania, and there is still a bronze plaque over the entrance to the clinic in College Hall, marking the event and place. Beyond that plaque and beyond Sarason's (1958) attention to Witmer as a clinician, Witmer's work has been largely forgotten. Recently some have begun to note Witmer's contributions. Because the spirit of his work is so modern, we hope this brief introduction will lead to renewed interest in what he had to offer.

Witmer's influence

Witmer, Philadelphia born and educated in private schools, was a graduate of the University of Pennsylvania and a law student, although he left the Penn law school after a year. In the philosophy department he came into contact with G. S. Fullerton, and with James McKeen Cattell, who encouraged him to study at Leipzig for his Ph.D. On his return to the United States he was made Director of the Laboratory of Psychology at the University of Pennsylvania, succeeding Cattell, who was called to Columbia the previous year. It is likely that Witmer took some of his interest in the study of individual differences from Cattell.

Witmer was evidently a very complex person. He was an intellectual, he was interested in dangerous sports, and he enlisted in the Spanish American War to find out how he would behave in battle. Though he was outspokenly liberal in his political opinions, he lived as an aristocrat, becoming more and more selective of friends until some thought of him as a distant, solitary figure. In his later years, colleagues and students said he was disorganized and erratic. He was never accorded the professional recognition he deserved, but those who knew him in his earlier days spoke of him reverently as an individual, as a clinician, and as an intellectual (Brotemarkle, 1931).

It remains a problem to understand why Witmer's contributions continue to receive so little attention by professional psychologists. A perusal of the *Psychological Review* after 1896 did not turn up a single reference to Witmer's work, nor even any notice of the beginning of his journal. It is possible that Witmer's influence was not more acknowledged because of academic inbreeding. Many of his students, Twitmeyer, Miller, Viteles, Brotemarkle, Murphy, and Phillips, stayed on with the clinic or with the University of Pennsylvania psychology department. Many of these men developed branching interests which were encouraged by Witmer. Thus Viteles went into vocational guidance and then industrial psychology; Twitmeyer developed reading problems as a specialty; while Brotemarkle concentrated on college personnel problems. A number of his other students worked in the Philadelphia area, so that many of his students may simply have not been in a position to carry the word far afield. In later years, some potential students were lost because of an aversion to the lack of validation of Witmer's clinical methods.

Witmer's influence is vastly underrated today. Certainly after the publication of *The Psychological Clinic*, beginning in 1906, his influence must have been fairly widespread. Witmer was aware of his lack of recognition, and in a paper written in 1925 he complained that he had been given that most sincere tribute, imitation, but too often without acknowledgement (Witmer, 1931).

The Phipps Psychiatric Clinic at Johns Hopkins, for example, operated a special class with a focus on the educational process as the prime mode of therapy. Campbell (1919), one of the noted figures in American psychiatry, speaks in glowing terms of the effects of this special class program in reducing truancy, in reducing appearances before the Juvenile Court, in changing the children's personal habits, and in opening the children's parents to additional help and education. The program is highly reminiscent of Witmer's special classes at the University of Pennsylvania (Witmer, 1911), but Campbell's article does not mention Witmer.

Given the development of clinics in subsequent years, his complaints had some justice. By 1934 there were at least 85 psychoeducational clinics which were university affiliated, although likely to be located in schools of education and not in psychology departments. These were engaged in training and in service, helping to effect the educational, vocational, or social adjustment of children from pre-schoolers to high school students (Witty & Theman, 1934). One can also safely estimate that many psychological services connected with public schools, including special class programs, were influenced directly or indirectly by Witmer's clinic.

Shakow (1948) and Watson (1953) have suggested that Witmer's narrow experimental orientation and his emphasis on the cognitive aspect of retardation to the exclusion of psychodynamic considerations led him away from what came to be the main thrust of clinical interest. Witmer did emphasize the experimental method. He published *Analytical Psychology* (Witmer, 1902), a laboratory manual of experiments in perception, sensation, attention, memory, reaction time, and similar topics, after he started the clinic. Even his clinical thinking is couched in experimental terms. Members of the Psychonomic Society, a group who separated themselves from the label "psychologist" because of the applied connotations of that word, will be interested in knowing that Witmer (1931) used the term "psychonomics" in 1925. He defined psychonomic as denoting that which is in conformity with a fundamental or universal law of thought and he claimed that the clinical method had a basically psychonomic orientation in that it was dedicated toward developing scientific explanations of the full range of behavior, not only the abnormal. As we shall see, he conceived the therapeutic interaction, as a form of experiment. The method of diagnostic teaching consisted of the development and testing of hypotheses about the factors involved in the educational retardation of each individual case.

While it is true that Witmer made no use of psychoanalytic concepts per se (he acknowledges some degree of intellectual indebtedness to Freud [Witmer, 1931]), an examination of his case studies cannot fail to reveal his understanding of character development and ego functioning in highly sophisticated terms. Although he did not employ the language of psychoanalysis, Witmer was keenly aware of familial etiology and of interpersonal influences upon intellectual functioning. His orientation was far from a static one.

Witmer was a highly sophisticated clinician who employed methods which repay study, especially today in an age in which the clinician is turning toward the educational setting as a means of dealing with the problems of emotionally disturbed children. Witmer developed effective approaches for a variety of disturbed children, not only intellectual retardates. His case studies, his discussion of the clinical method, and his insistence on considering the qualitative aspects of performance in addition to the quantitative distribution of test scores, in no way supports the view that he was a narrow experimentalist. Witmer's neglect is a real historical mystery.

A partial explanation is suggested by some evidence that Witmer's temperament and personal style fostered the neglect accorded to his work. In 1908, he attacked both William James and Hugo Munsterberg for their lack of devotion to laboratory experimentation and scientific method. James was interested in such non-experimental topics as psychical phenomena, while Munsterberg abandoned his interests in laboratory experimentation and moved in strongly applied directions. In fact, Munsterberg is considered the father of applied psychology (Boring, 1957; Roback, 1964). Witmer's attack (Roback, 1961) on both James and Munsterberg was so strong that the latter wanted to lodge a formal protest with the American Psychological Association.

James wrote a letter to Munsterberg in an attempt to dissuade him from responding to Witmer's attack (James, 1926, II, 320). Why Witmer should feel so vehemently about the interests of those two men is unclear. Viteles (personal communication), who recalls that Witmer was also at odds with Cattell, has suggested that Witmer's attack upon several past presidents of APA, combined with his aloofness, may have contributed to his relative neglect by the field. Roback (1961; 1964) suggests the same.

Witmer did serve on American Psychological Association Committees after 1908, but in a world so small that the entire membership of the American Psychological Association could meet in a single lecture room in College Hall at the University of Pennsylvania, personal style might well have had an important effect on the reception given a man's ideas. Someone has wisely said that a cause ought not to be judged by its first adherents.

origins of the clinic

As a university student, Witmer taught English in a college preparatory academy. There he encountered a young man who was preparing for college entrance, but notably deficient in the use of English. Witmer tutored him, and succeeded in helping him sufficiently so that he was able to enter the University of Pennsylvania. There Witmer again encountered him, this time as a student in his college course. The young man, with great difficulty, managed to graduate from a professional school, but Witmer felt that the young man might have struggled less had he had special training in his earlier years.

The case which actually began the clinic was brought to Witmer by an elementary school principal who was taking psychology courses at the University of Pennsylvania. She challenged Witmer to apply the New Psychology to diagnose and to cure a spelling deficiency. Witmer was struck that the science of psychology had absolutely nothing to say about spelling; and spelling failure was, after all, a deficiency of memory, a subject about which psychology was supposed to have furnished authoritative knowledge. Witmer wrote, "It appeared to me that if psychology was worth anything to me or to others it should be able to assist the efforts of a teacher in a retarded case of this kind." Beginning with that case, in the spring of 1896, Witmer started seeing a few children several hours each week to attempt to train them to overcome some specific disabilities in subject matter.

By December, 1896, Witmer (1897) had developed a farsighted plan for "practical work" in psychology directed toward the investigation of mental development in school children, as manifested in "mental and moral retardation," the investigation to be conducted by means of clinical and statistical methods. He urged the development of a clinic, supplemented by a hospital school for the treatment of such children, and he proposed that the clinic be used for the training of teachers, social workers, and physicians. His final goal was that of training students for a new profession, that of the psychological expert who would examine and treat mentally and morally retarded children and who would work in connection with the school system.

the clinical method and the community

The term "clinical" was employed to indicate the method Witmer felt he was using. The clinical psychologist was interested in the individual child, and examined and proposed treatment to promote the next steps in the child's mental and physical development. Witmer quite clearly saw that the clinical psychologist operated as a scientist to the degree that he saw himself attempting to discover cause and effect relationships in applying his remedies to children suffering from some form of retardation. He did not restrict clinical to mean the study of the abnormal only. "For the methods of clinical psychology are necessarily invoked wherever the status of an individual mind is determined by observation and experiment and pedagogical treatment applied to effect a change, i.e., the development of such individual mind. Whether the subject be a child or an adult, the examination and treatment may be conducted and their results expressed in terms of the clinical method" (Witmer, 1906, p. 9).

Earlier, Witmer thought that clinical psychology would be closely allied with medicine, but by 1906 his position had changed considerably:

Although clinical psychology is closely related to medicine, it is quite as closely related to sociology and to pedagogy.

The school room, the Juvenile Court, and the streets are a larger laboratory of psychology. An abundance of material for scientific study fails to be utilized, because the interest of psychologists is elsewhere engaged, and those in constant touch with the actual phenomena do not possess the training necessary to make their experience and observation of scientific value.

While the field of clinical psychology is to some extent occupied by the physician, especially the psychiatrist, and while I expect to rely in a great measure upon the educator and the social worker for the more important contributions to this branch of psychology, it is nevertheless true that none of these has quite the training necessary for this kind of work. For that matter, neither has the psychologist, unless he has acquired this training from other sources than the usual course of instruction in psychology. In fact, we must look forward to the training of men to a new profession which will be exercised more particularly in connection with educational problems, but for which the training of the psychologist will be a prerequisite (pp. 7–8).

Witmer's 1906 statement is surprisingly relevant to the contemporary community mental health movement, and the organization of his clinic with its close relationship to the local educational setting is also worthy of note. In its early days the clinic was not an institution separate from the schools, but was closely tied in with them. When Witmer read a paper to the APA in 1896 (Witmer, 1897) announcing a program in practical work in psychology, he included the following two points. First, he wanted to develop special or upgraded training classes for children who were backward or physically defective. These classes were to be organized under the control of the city school authorities, but to be in "harmonious and effective relationship" with the department of psychology. Second, he insisted that the program include instruction in psychology for public school teachers. He felt they needed, above all else, courses in the practical study of children.

Witmer was close to and was widely respected by educators in the Philadelphia area and elsewhere. He helped to establish special classes in the public schools and wrote an extensive monograph on special classes with Van Sickle and Ayres (1911). The Philadelphia system used his term "orthogenic" for its classes for backward children for many years. Witmer lists a number of school superintendents and supervisors who were closely associated with him in the clinic. The principal who brought the second case to him is later listed as one of the lecturers in a summer institute given in 1907, along with Corn-man, a principal, and Bryant and Twitmeyer, both superintendents of schools. Another teacher, Mary Marvin, was associated with Witmer from the very beginning. These were more than summer institutes con-descendingly offered for teachers. Classes for observation and experi-mentation were conducted as part of the clinic teaching and therapy program (Witmer, 1911). They provided a situation in which clinical psychologists and teachers participated completely in the training of each other, a situation rarely found today, and one that the community mental health movement seeks to establish. This influence was con-tinued through the many education students who took his courses.

diagnosis

The literature does not contain any really good description of Witmer's clinic in terms of its intake policy, referral sources, and other operational matters. During the first ten years of the clinic, Witmer did almost all of the psychological examination himself. Cases were brought to him from a variety of sources, including school people, the visiting nurse service, and later from private sources. His proce-dure included examination by medical specialists for neurological disorders, for possible defects of vision or audition, even for diseased tonsils and adenoids. Apparently Witmer made use of an extensive battery of psychological tests, including the Witmer Formboard and the Witmer Cylinders, tests standardized by his students over the course of the years. While Witmer emphasized the individual, he was a pioneer in insisting upon obtaining adequate normative data for his tests. In later years, the Binet was used. A variety of tests of memory, attention, sensory acuity, and association ability were employed.

Witmer emphasized most strongly that test scores revealed mini-mal information. He taught at a very early date that a test score could be composed of a vast variety of correct and incorrect performances, and that such a score hid the details of the individual's performances.

He imbued his students with the notion that each individual should be examined carefully and that the qualitative data are the most important to obtain. Where one person would see only a failure in an incorrect response, Witmer was constantly searching for signs of intelligence in the way in which the individual went about handling the task set before him. Many of the case studies do not even report I.Q.'s.

diagnostic teaching—a method of therapy

Witmer's contributions to psychodiagnostics are probably of less immediate relevance than his contributions to therapy. Witmer worked with a concept of diagnostic education. He felt one could not finally make a diagnosis until one had attempted to teach a child something. For Witmer, diagnostic teaching was an experimental method by which one attempted to understand the individual case by systematically devising educational techniques which would test hypotheses about the factors which cause or maintain the particular condition. He laid stress upon continuing diagnosis, made through a prolonged period of educational treatment with every step determined by whatever was known about the child to that point, and modified as more was learned. Repeated measurement of actual achievement validated the correctness of the ongoing diagnosis and the effectiveness of the remedial treatment.

An attempt to teach a child something beyond his known level of performance, carried out consistently several times a week for periods up to a year or more, and carried to the point where the teaching could be continued at home or in school, under clinic supervision, represented the essence of the method. Even in the later years when the direct ties to the public schools were no longer strong, clinic personnel always tried to involve teachers and principals in the clinic's work. Two-way communication was maintained and teachers would sometimes be asked to come to the clinic to participate in the examination of the child. Students preparing to do clinic teaching were sent to the schools to do classroom observations, and they frequently would carry out clinic teaching in school or hospital settings (Viteles, personal communication).

Clinic teaching was a primary mode of outpatient therapy. Witmer always attempted to assess the abilities a child possessed, abilities which could be employed in helping him toward some preferred pattern of adaptation. For Witmer always sought answers to the question of what could be done next to help the child to take yet another step—to increase his ability to learn.

the hospital school

The hospital school, a facility vital to Witmer's approach, was first established in 1907. The hospital school was a residential center providing medical care, nursing care, and education primarily to private patients on a fee basis, but exceptionally interesting cases were admitted with little or no fee. Children were admitted for diagnostic purposes, that is, an attempt was made to train the children. They would stay anywhere from a few days up to a year or more. Training extended to education and self-care. However, the hospital school was not just an inpatient institution. In some instances the children were taught at the classes held at the University of Pennsylvania Clinic, and in some instances schooling took place on the grounds of the hospital school. In addition, children were often enrolled in local public school classes (Witmer, 1908a) and the trainer (Witmer's term for the hospital school supervisor, originally a nurse) stayed in very close touch with the public school teacher. Witmer was clearly aware of the problem of returning the child to the community and he acted to reduce the discontinuity between the institutional and the normal setting.

therapeutic methods

The trainers had fairly sophisticated psychotherapeutic techniques at their command, but they used them in the natural setting, as the problems arose. For example, in one case (Witmer, 1908b) outbursts of rage, largely related to the jealousy and competitiveness of one child with another, were treated by the trainer and other attendants, who discussed the problem with the boy over and over again. At one point, the patient was given the task of playing a game with another child without losing his temper. When he accomplished the task, he happily reported the fact to the trainer. The trainer helped him to label his undesirable behavior as a "mean mood," and to some extent the child seemed to try to control his "mean mood" to win the trainer's approval.

The assistant trainer interpreted his behavior to him as self-defeating, the discussion taking place immediately, and in the situation in which the behavior occurred. The assistant trainer pointed out how his "mean moods" caused him to be shunned by others and the staff generally held out the expectation that he should and would begin to control himself better.

That this consistent treatment had an effect is seen in an incident in which the boy was ordered to leave the dinner table to wash his hands. He got up, pouted angrily, and said, "I won't come back!" However, he washed his hands and when he came back, he explained that, "I nearly got mad, but I just said to myself 'I will control my temper.'" The reader may be interested in comparing the technique in treating this boy with Redl's life space interview (Redl, 1966).

While Witmer was not much of a theoretician, an examination of his cases and those of his students suggests that he frequently operated with the hypothesis that a low level of frustration tolerance, accompanied by a lack of demand from a parental figure that a child learn to tolerate the tension of frustration, was a causative element in retardation. In one article Witmer wrote: "I believe that the home and school, chiefly through neglect of discipline, permit the minds of many children to remain undeveloped during the formative period. The discipline that is required is not merely that which makes for obedience. It is the discipline of work and strenuous effort, the discipline that trains the memory, the will, the attention and forms habits of work which permit children to assume progressively more difficult tasks" (Witmer, 1908–1909b, p. 158).

In many of the cases he describes, both those with whom he worked himself, and those who were treated by teachers or trainers at his hospital school, he seemed to place great reliance on the consistent, firm demand that the individual do what was required of him. He was not insensitive to problems stemming from anxiety, however. Witmer's indomitable will is admirably depicted in a number of the orthogenic cases described by Witmer or his students.

Albert (Parker, 1917) for example, was described by his mother as "lazy; he answers in any fashion to avoid thinking. He is gluttonous, sluggish, indifferent and thoughtless." At fourteen and a half, his academic achievement level was judged to be no higher than fourth grade. He could add, subtract, multiply, and divide by rote, but he could not solve problems which required even simple addition or multiplication. He knew little or nothing of geography or history or current events. He read at a sixth grade level and spelled at a fifth grade level, but comprehension was quite poor. He could not retain the plot of a movie and could not handle formal grammar, but he could compose stories rather well. In Witmer's school, observers described Albert as mentally lazy, not liking to work, and playing or bluffing his way through lessons. His attention wandered continuously, and he had neither self-control nor any ability to work independently. He seemed to need someone at his side continuously to drive him or coax him. He drove his teachers to distraction by making random, irrelevant comments and by restless fidgeting and inattentiveness. Albert behaved in this manner for five months under the care of two teachers who were unable to cope with him.

Five months later, Albert encountered Mrs. G., who was employed as a housemother.[1] She was described as big, a Viking of a woman with a tremendous physique. She was a woman of "dynamic will, a will of immense energy to attempt the impossible, of extraordinary power to dominate the mind and behavior of those with whom she lived." Immediately on meeting Albert, for reasons described very picturesquely, Mrs. G. set herself to tame and transform him. Every aspect of his life was put under a firm, demanding regime. He was forced to wash, to diet, to eat slowly and with good manners, to stop annoying children and adults in the house, and to dress tastefully and cleanly. He was bullied into exercising and into performing manual labor. The following incident gives something of the flavor of Mrs. G.'s treatment of Albert.

---

[1] Witmer, one gathers, was no respecter of academic degrees. In this case and in others, teachers, nurses, and housemothers apparently played an important role in the therapy of children in the clinic and in the hospital school. In this case (Parker, 1917) Albert's relationship with Mrs. G. went far beyond anything which would be tolerated, much less encouraged in most contemporary residential treatment centers. Witmer said that some of the best trainers he knew had no formal background in special education.

One hot afternoon in August, Albert had been sent to rake
leaves from the shrubbery over the edge of the hill above
the creek. Presently, he came into the cool of the living
room, mopping his face.

"I can't rake down there any more, Mrs. G. There's a
yellow jacket's nest there."

Mrs. G., unfamiliar with English, thought that "yellow
jackets" were "little yellow birds." She pointed to the door
with a long arm and compelling finger, and her answer was
a single guttural monosyllable:

"R-r-r-r-rake!"

Albert raked. After a little, he returned to receive precisely the same answer:

"R-r-r-r-rake!"

A third time he came back and still Mrs. G. had for him but
one word: "R-r-r-r-rake!"

And Albert raked!

There was a magnificent thoroughness in Albert's subjuga-
tion that, in spite of his resentment, bred in him a respect
for the forces that had so mastered him.

That such treatment in which one insistently demanded discipline
was concurred in by Witmer is indicated by the following excerpt in
which Witmer himself prescribed for Albert.

Inside the classroom as well as outside, Albert was subjected to a new regime of vigorous discipline. During the
first few days in June, Dr. Witmer himself worked with him.
For once in his life the nervous wriggling boy did not move
a finger. For the first time, he sat at his desk absolutely
quiet.

Dr. Witmer, from his examination, concluded that Albert had been pushed too far ahead in geography, history
and arithmetic. Because of the picture of mental confusion
which he presented, and the conspicuous defect in persistent
concentration of attention, Dr. Witmer decided that some
weeks of mental discipline must precede any attempt to give
Albert additional information. Thoroughness and precision
were the qualities which must be developed in him by the

summer's work. Albert had, as Dr. Witmer remarked, a mind that "skims." He must be given tasks requiring exactness and completeness—tasks through which he could not skim. Above everything else, there was to be no "speeding up," no attempt to cover ground. Every single point must be known exactly and thoroughly. The teacher's motto, like General Grant's must be, "I'll fight it out on this line if it takes all summer."

Dr. Witmer's outline for Albert's work in the next few months, therefore included:

(1) The memorizing with absolute accuracy of the definitions in Webster's Abridged Dictionary, of words taken from Rice's Rational Spelling Book—Fourth Year—a very few words each day.

(2) The memorizing, word for word, of the illustrative sentences in Rice's Speller containing the words studied.

(3) The composition of original sentences containing the words studied.

(4) Drill in penmanship in which precision must be rigidly insisted upon.

(5) Simple stories like those in Aesop's Fables and Baldwin's Fifty Famous Stories; read and reread every word until every sentence was read with absolute accuracy.

(6) Oral and written reproduction of each story until he could reproduce the content of what he had read in a logical and comprehensive manner.

(7) The writing of solutions of simple arithmetic problems, to exercise his reasoning faculty within the limits of his very elementary comprehension.

With this outline for work, Dr. Witmer handed Albert over to a vigorous young woman whose discipline was more adequate to the situation than that of the man who had first taught him. Dr. Witmer, too, continued his close supervision of the work throughout the summer and from time to time took over the actual teaching for one or two hours a day.

Miss B. carried out the prescribed program energetically and faithfully. She made Albert work in the classroom, and what is more remarkable, she made him work by himself, outside the classroom an hour and a half in the afternoon, and sometimes an hour in the evening. To accomplish this, she had, at first, literally to follow him around with his work and force him to it. "There is nothing in the world," she wrote, "that he minds more than to have to sit down and learn a thing alone." . . .

Each day, Miss B. gave Albert eight definitions to learn. Any that he did not know he had to write ten times after dinner. This penalty was invariable and inescapable. During the first week, or so, an hour or two after dinner went into the tiresome task of writing and rewriting definitions. This work began on the first day of June. It was the twenty-first day of July before Albert was able to recite correctly in the morning recitation the eight definitions assigned for the day (Parker, Vol. II, 1917).

The remainder of the case study goes on to describe Albert's further encounters with Mrs. G., his continued treatment in the hospital school, and his later adjustment at a preparatory school. Albert was considerably changed, although he continued to have a variety of problems, and by no means did well at school. However, he was now functioning at something approaching his age level, and was no longer so obnoxious that he was thrown out of his regular school.

The excerpt from a rather long and fascinating case study reflects Witmer's method of diagnostic teaching quite well. On the basis of tests and observations, Witmer came to certain conclusions about the characteristics of Albert's mind. He did not focus on his infantile regressive behavior, nor did he concern himself with the provocative hostility shown by this boy. His attack on the problem was quite direct. The boy's infantile character **was** treated by persistent demands that he meet new standards. The adults who were successful with him were forceful, and overpowering in their determination that he comply, but there is no indication they were ever punitive toward him. Similarly, Witmer's approach to Albert's educational deficiencies was direct.

While one may question the faculty psychology which Witmer seemed to employ, it is clear that he was trying to develop work habits and a level of frustration tolerance, in keeping with his theoretical views that some instances of retardation were due to a lack of discipline in work and in exerting strenuous effort to overcome frustration. Witmer did not concern himself with any possible psychodynamics in the learn-

ing inhibition, but rather he attacked it directly, and used the indica-
tions the boy could learn as diagnostic signs that he could be taught
still more. There is no evidence in this case that any other symptoms
developed with the direct attack on his learning problem. The reader
may compare Witmer's approach to the education of the emotionally
disturbed child with the similar method found most effective by Haring
and Phillips (1962) in their careful study of various approaches to the
education of the emotionally disturbed child.

In an article entitled "Diagnostic Education" (Witmer, 1917),
Witmer offers a case study in which the method of diagnostic education
is illustrated in pure form. The case is remarkable not only for its
achievement, but also because it illustrates Witmer's indomitable spirit,
his willingness to try, and his desire not to accept a diagnosis implying
hopelessness. The case also illustrates methods which both teach and
diagnose at the same time, and it demonstrates his ingenuity and sensitivity in interpreting qualitative aspects of performance in any situation. While the case is not very long in the original article, it is presented somewhat dryly, and we shall omit unnecessary detail for the
sake of easing the reader's task.

> The case is of a boy, two years and seven months old[2] at
> the time treatment began, who was initially diagnosed by
> Witmer and by an independent authority as feebleminded.
> The child was born of normal, healthy parents. . . . His
> birth and development were uneventful until six months of
> age, when he had an attack of whooping cough. From then
> on, if placed on the floor he stayed put. If he fell on his face,
> he lay there until picked up. He made no effort to reach
> normally attractive objects, but spent most of his time in
> bed unresponsive and indifferent. He crept at 26 months
> only after his knees were moved by someone else. His walk
> at 31 months was still wobbly. He could not negotiate
> stairs. Given an object, he would hold it, staring at it by the
> hour. The hair on the back of his head was rubbed off and
> he had self-inflicted sores about his mouth and ears. He went
> into a violent temper tantrum if anyone attempted to take

[2] This case is probably "Donnie" (Witmer, 1919), reprinted in Sarason and Doris
(1968). To supplement his understanding of Witmer's approach, the reader is urged
to consult that case report.

anything away from him or move him. He said only the words "kitty" or "daddy," but could respond to the question, "What does the crow say?" by responding, "caw, caw." Language comprehension seemed limited to pointing out a few of his facial parts when asked. He made no effort to imitate actions and did not seem to look at things. A lighted match passed through his field of vision seemed to startle him. He would hold a book and turn its pages and could hold a watch to his ear and say "tick tock." He did not feed himself and was still in diapers. Witmer undertook his training only because of the earnest pleading of the boy's parents. His first response was that the boy was feeble-minded.

The following paragraphs are quotations from Witmer's account of his educational approach with this boy.

". . . I put before him the formboard consisting of eleven blocks of different shapes, each of which had its corresponding receptacle. He would not make the slighest effort even to pick a block to put it back in place. I then tried him with the peg board, a board of 36 holes into which a corresponding number of pegs of the same size and shape can be placed. He could not imitate my action of putting a peg in its hole. He could not put a peg in the hole even when I placed the peg in his hand. I had to hold his hand, guide it to the hole and place it in position, but after having done this once, he put five or six pegs in successively. In all he put in fifteen before I stopped, although after the first six he put in each successive peg only when I said emphatically, "Put in another peg." I never knew him to fill the board with 36 pegs as the result of a general command. His attention appeared to wander and he always desisted. In this his behavior was exactly like that of a chimpanzee whom I taught, though not with the same ease, to put pegs in a board. *Subsequent events proved that the reason he objected to putting 36 pegs into the board was because this action bored him, and not because he lacked persistent powers of attention.*" (Italics added)

Witmer goes on to discuss how he taught the child to work at the form board in the same fashion, at first by manipulating his hand and later by ordering him to place the forms. Witmer gradually gave him more and more forms which the boy had to discriminate until by the seventh day of training, the boy could place six forms in their proper insert without error. Witmer notes the boy's coordination was good. Within two weeks, the boy placed 11 insets without error in 85 seconds. From this experience, Witmer concluded the child had a retentive memory, good imagery, good analytic attentiveness and that he could be interested in a relatively difficult problem. As the boy's interest lagged in the form board Witmer gave him practice for several weeks on a more difficult performance task. Within three weeks the child mastered the task, and again lost all interest in it.

Witmer then decided to teach the child to discriminate the letters of the alphabet. "On April 17th I taught him the letter B, using for the purpose the large wooden block letter, saying, "This is B. Put B on the chair." In the afternoon he had forgotten it. After three separate periods of instruction he could pick out A, B, and C. He was asked to name them at the same time but would only name B. Some things you can force a child to do, but some things you cannot. I could compel him to pick out these letters but I could not compel him to name them, so I had to tempt him with new letters and new words. I got him to say "V" on one trial by dragging out the "V" sound. He loved the sound of the letter and the feel of making it, but it took nearly two weeks to get him to say "F."

Within three weeks time, the child had learned to pick out all twenty-six letters, although he still confused M, N, and W. There was an interruption of one month, but in July Witmer began working to test his ability to learn combinations of letters, in effect to learn to spell. He began by giving him the three letters of the word cat, and he was told to arrange them in the proper order. Within one month, he learned to arrange the letters of the words *cat, boy* and *pig* when these were presented to him. By August, he learned to arrange the letters for *cat* and *boy* when given the six letters, and he could spell *cat* or *bat* on command when given the letters BCAT.

"When a child is being taught, I always insist that he shall be taught at attention, on his toes as it were. Work is work and play is play. I even find that the same person cannot both teach and play with a child. Regularity of work is also an essential. The interruption of a few days usually means a great waste of time before the child's attention can be regained and held. In the early part of September, he showed a great gain when after an interruption of four or five days, he buckled down to work again without waste of effort.

Beginning September 8th, words were printed on pieces of paper and passed to him to read. He began to read words by first spelling them. On September the 11th the words, "I see a cat," were put before him and he was asked to read the sentence. *Dog, pig,* etc., were on September 14th substituted for the word *cat.* By September 19th he could read the sentences, "A man can see me." "A boy can see a dog." On September 21st I tested his newly acquired ability by putting Monroe's primer into his hand for the first time. He read, "I can see a man. A man ran. A cat can see a rat." It was done haltingly, but it showed that from this time on the acquisition of reading was to be only a matter of drill. He can now both spell and sound words and will probably be graduated into the first reader by the first of next June.

I do not care whether this boy can read or not. I have had him taught reading because it was the best way to engage his interest and train his attention, imagination and memory. He liked it, so far as anyone can be said to like work. Intellectual work I call this, and intellectual work, I say without hesitation, is an advantageous mental and hygienic stimulus to any boy of three years of age" (Witmer, 1917, pp. 77–78).

His achievement in teaching a child of less than three to read is itself remarkable, but his undertaking this task with a child who was probably psychotic and who appeared to be grossly defective is even more remarkable. The case reveals Witmer's sensitivity to qualitative cues, his ability to see the future potential in behavior rather than its pathology, and his infinite patience and persistence in working with the child. His procedures were planned at every step, and progressed from teaching the simplest discriminations to developing complex sequential discriminations. He very carefully took him step-by-step, in a sequence which reminds one very much of the concepts of the teaching machine. He started with the simplest step, and moved him gradually into more complicated material, using the boy's intrinsic interest in the tasks and Witmer's social approval as the sources of reinforcement.

the perfectibility of man

Witmer seemed to share with other great educators a basic belief in the perfectibility of man (Mensh, 1966). The great educators accept the principle that each individual has within him the potential for growth, and their methods are directed toward eliciting that potential. In his clinical work, Witmer started with the assumption that a child could learn, despite apparent pathology, despite the apparent hopelessness of a situation. One can argue that an integral part of Witmer's clinical methodology was an unswerving faith that if he maintained a firm expectation that his child could learn, that child would learn. On a broader level, Witmer saw that if diagnostic education could produce such dramatic results with children who were clearly retarded, it held broad promise for the education of normal children. Witmer's outlook can be compared with Montessori's. She started her work with retarded children. When she taught them sufficiently to pass normal school examinations, she concluded that something was lacking in the teaching methods in the public schools which permitted her retarded children to equal the performance of normal children (Montessori, 1964).

Witmer began with an attempt to apply the scientific psychology of the day to the practical problem of education, because he felt that both psychology and education would be benefited. In keeping with the reform spirit of his day, he viewed his approach as a means of changing public education to make it more responsive to individual needs. He did not start out with the assumption that the people were inferior or sick because they did not respond to the current teaching methods. Rather he started with the assumption that it would be possible to find ways of teaching which would take into account the characteristics of the people being taught. In contrast to psychotherapeutic approaches which both implicitly and explicitly demand that the individual acknowledge his sickness before he can be helped, Witmer's educational approach seemed to assume that it was indeed possible for any individual to respond to a proper set of conditions. If we wished to put the difference in classical terms, we might say the psychotherapist is concerned with "original sin" in his emphasis on the sickness of the individual. He believes there is some evil within the individual which must be exorcised or controlled before the individual can achieve a state of grace. Witmer might be said to be emphasizing the concept that each man contains the "spark of the divine," that if one expects a man to be good then that good will be elicited. We believe it is no accident that Witmer emphasized such a conception when he did, nor was it an accident that he started with school problems. Both his basic philosophy and the social problems he undertook to correct were products of ongoing social change. We shall see similar viewpoints and similar therapeutic philosophies when we examine some of the other helping agencies which evolved during the same period.

In more immediately practical terms, it seems to us that Witmer's case studies and his educational approaches have much to say to those seeking new ways of helping. At the very least his achievements should lead to a reexamination of the assumption that any approach other than the psychotherapeutic is superficial. Moreover, the focus of Witmer's clinic gives the field of clinical psychology a much different view of the traditional. Those currently interested in educational and community oriented approaches are continuing the earliest tradition of the field, a tradition Lightner Witmer helped to establish, and one in which he made substantive contributions.

5

the settlement house movement—
bridge between worlds

If history provides any model for the contemporary community mental health movement, it is the settlement house of the pre-World War I period. The settlement house developed as a means of coping with the social disorganization induced by rapid industrialization, urbanization, and immigration in the period following the Civil War. Its purpose was to promote the organic unity of society by reducing the distance between social classes; it accomplished its purpose by providing an institutionalized form of help at the very point at which there seemed to be the greatest disintegration of the social order. At its best, the settlement house initiated action to achieve sweeping changes in what was then viewed as the basic social causes of personal misery.

The early settlement house workers were highly educated young people with a bent toward social action. At their best, they created an exciting intellectual environment within the settlement houses in which all manner of people could meet and freely exchange ideas. In addition to their helping purpose, the early settlement houses, often university affiliated, were designed as living laboratories for the "sociologists" of that day. In fact, they were the means whereby an enormous amount of social research was accomplished, the research providing the basis for programmatic efforts at sweeping social change.

Far from being mindless do-gooders, the best of the settlement house workers were social scientists intimately involved with the problems of the real world. Theirs was an effort to understand their society in order to make it into a more effective democracy, one in which their belief in the perfectibility of man could be realized.

early antecedents

The settlement house in the United States was a direct outgrowth of a movement established earlier in England. The industrial revolution in England preceded that in the United States by more than a half century and the social problems it created called forth a new humanitarianism early exemplified by Robert Owen. He experimented with providing good pay, enlightened working conditions, a healthy family life, recreation, education, and a sense of community among his workers.[1] Owen's experiments were not widely adopted, and as industrialization progressed the lot of the working man worsened. Against the backdrop of social unrest which erupted in revolutions on the Continent in the mid-19th century, philosophers, economists, historians, and social critics developed new ideas concerning the social order. Carlyle, John Stuart Mill, Marx and Engels, and later Tolstoy propounded new views of society based on concepts concerning the distribution of wealth and the responsibilities of different groups in society toward each other. Charles Dickens' novels and stories were instrumental in bringing the plight of the poor to the attention of the upper classes and in paving the way for a variety of reforms.

In England, theological schools and churches developed the concept of the kingdom of God on earth, a concept embodied in the philosophy of the Christian Socialists. The Christian Socialists early and actively supported the developing labor movement by their writings, by fund raising, and by advising labor leaders. Experience with the labor movement led the Christian Socialists to feel that higher

[1] The history and the social factors of Owen's experiments might well be the subject of renewed interest of those concerned with projects in community development.

education for the working man was an absolute necessity. A volunteer teaching staff of young university men who had shown themselves to be intellectually distinguished came to the fore and established a highly successful teaching enterprise in working-class neighborhoods, a forerunner of the university extension program.

After 1860, men who had been involved in the Christian Socialist movement, or who had supported its tenets, came into power at the major universities. These men—Matthew Arnold, the poet and critic, and John Ruskin, in fine arts, at Oxford, and Charles Kingsley, in history, and Frederick Maurice, professor of moral philosophy, at Cambridge—critical of the cultural poverty of their time, called for the wide dissemination of the best of knowledge and culture in order to prepare the foundations of a true democracy.

As early as the 1860's educated, upper-class individuals started to live among workingmen in England, just as in Russia, under the influence of Tolstoy, Russian nobility attempted to share the lives of the peasants. Men such as Edward Denison and Arnold Toynbee, with the support and approbation of their professors, began to comprehend and to voice some of the problems of working-class neighborhoods. Samuel Barnett, a minister, requested the vicarage of St. Jude's, Whitechapel, described as the "wretchedest" parish in the London diocese. Barnett's vicarage became a center for young Oxford men who were interested in serving.

Through his influence a university extension center was established in his parish. The center and its activities received wide publicity. Barnett planned to introduce a group of educated men as leaders in areas without constructive local leadership, where the hard facts of industrial life had led to disorganization. He proposed that a house be rented where university men could "settle" for an extended period of time, studying the life and the problems of a working-class neighborhood.[2] Barnett insisted that close personal acquaintance with the problems was an absolute prerequisite to intelligent public action and he warned that no helping scheme would have a chance of success unless it brought the helper and the helped into a friendly, mutually understanding relationship.

[2] Abell (1943) points out that the settlement house movement developed partly as a reaction to the Salvation Army, itself an outgrowth of a strong religious mission movement of the time. In England and in the United States, the Salvation Army with its military technique was characterized at first as vulgar and ridiculous and

Toynbee Hall, named for Arnold Toynbee, who had died young, was opened on Christmas Eve of 1884. Toynbee Hall became an important model for the American settlement house movement; Jane Addams, Stanton Coit, Robert Woods, Charles Zeublin, and many other leaders of the movement either visited or were in residence at Toynbee Hall in the years preceding their work in the United States (Woods, 1891; Woods & Kennedy, 1922; Barnett, 1950).

origins in America

The rise of an urban, industrial society in the United States in the years after the Civil War was accompanied by what seemed to be a lowered standard of living for the laborer, crowded houses and tenements, unemployment, vice, delinquency, misery, and illness. Each successive wave of immigrants displaced the last in occupying the poorest areas of cities. The rise of the labor movement, the appearance of radicals of various persuasions, and widespread strikes and riots in

---

was viewed as a threat to established religious groups. Originally based on a far-reaching plan for the rehabilitation of the poor, the Salvation Army was not merely an evangelical group with uniforms, cornets, soup kitchens, and street-corner revival meetings. General William Booth, its founder, proposed establishing a series of colonies to retrain men to self-sufficiency. The first step was an urban colony in which a man was to be given food, shelter, and work, in order that he develop a willingness to work and freedom from the "more repulsive habits." Once basic work skills and attitudes were developed the man was to be placed in a cooperative industrial-farm village where he was to develop habits of self-reliance and resourcefulness. When this degree of rehabilitation was achieved, he was to be sent to an overseas colony and given suitable land. This plan was actually put into effect in the United States, and by 1897 there were three "colonies," in California, Colorado, and Ohio, involving some two hundred inhabitants. The Salvation Army also developed a widespread network of residences, schools, orphan asylums, employment bureaus, legal aid societies, life insurance companies, day nurseries, halfway houses for prisoners, a youth corps, and similar services for the urban poor. The model provided by the Salvation Army as a community action and anti-poverty program deserves reexamination by the contemporary social scientist.

Stanton Coit, who established the first American settlement house, opens his book describing the neighborhood guild concept, by stating: "No one has yet accepted, in the full sense in which he meant it, General Booth's challenge to bring forward a better scheme than his for lifting the fallen classes of society into independence and prosperity" (Coit, 1891, p. 1). He is explicit in presenting the settlement concept, with its emphasis on neighborhood organization and self-help, as an alternative to the Salvation Army.

the 1870's and 1880's called attention to the social problems of the working class. Henry George, Jacob Riis, Lincoln Steffens, and others wrote about the vast abuses suffered by the working man under corrupt municipal governments and unrestrained private enterprise.

The churches also came under attack and were under pressure to change. As "foreigners" and Catholics came in, the American Protestant churches moved out to the suburbs. The churches began to find that the gospel of salvation and abstract theological issues were irrelevant to the problems of the day. One survey showed that less than 10 percent of the working men in any given area attended church with any regularity.

While most churchmen supported the status quo, as early as the 1870's some ministers severely criticized the business ethics of the day, and talked of making Christian principles work here and now. American ministers also spoke about the kingdom of God on earth. Out of the ferment grew the social gospel movement, in which ministers, seeing themselves as the lineal successors to the Old Testament prophets, felt it their social and moral responsibility to denounce wrong, to explain right, and to lead people to the realization of their duty.[3] The social gospel novels, maudlin stories with Horatio Alger-like plots, were extraordinarily popular and effective in directing the middle class toward their Christian duty to those less fortunate than themselves.[4] Many in the ministry took up the cause of the developing labor movement, and involved themselves in a variety of other reforms.

The period in which the social gospel movement developed was also a period in which the physical sciences developed great influence. Religious thinkers found themselves under pressure to integrate their traditional role as the interpreters of society's morality with materialistic science, with evolution, and with the new Biblical criticism. Christian sociology developed. The early academic sociologists were interested in social reform, and Christian sociologists saw it as their

[3] One can compare articles by Cox (1967) and Callahan (1967) on the need of contemporary American religion for social relevance and for social action. The terms of the arguments are startlingly similar to those advanced by the social gospel pioneers around the turn of the century.
[4] The settlements, the Juvenile Court, and other helping agencies made use of volunteers who seemed to be available in huge numbers. The volunteer movement of that day seems not to have been subjected to socio-historical study. It should be, partly because it was a helping movement of sizeable proportion which was truly embedded in the community, and partly because the experience at that time might serve as a guide in understanding the present-day corps of volunteers.

mission to determine scientifically the principles of social organization and social conduct which would best promote social welfare and the ethical life. In the divinity schools of the great universities, through courses in social ethics and sociology and through an emphasis on field studies, religious thinkers influenced a whole generation of young men who then went out into the world to implement the concepts they had learned.

The need of the Protestant churches for new methods to attract the workingman led to the growth of the institutional church, the religious settlement, and the religious mission. The pattern of the institutional church was the YMCA and the Salvation Army. These were free, always open, and located in working-class neighborhoods.[5] Some of the institutional churches eventually evolved into non-sectarian settlements, but more importantly, the ministry of the social gospel made it possible and even necessary for the educated youths of the day to enter into helping and reform roles (Hopkins, 1940; Abell, 1943; Miller & Miller, 1962).

By the 1880's books such as Henry George's *Progress and Poverty* and the works of Marx and Engels appeared in print. New thought in economics and diverse views in philosophy, political science, sociology, and anthropology were advocated in the universities (Curti, 1951; Goldman, 1956). Spurred by their professors to be critical of the social order, intrigued by the philosophy of self-sacrifice propounded by Tolstoy and Ruskin, told that the source of wealth of the nation was "tainted," desirous of achieving a natural democracy, thoughtful students who saw only conventional careers for themselves were placed in conflict.[6] The settlements were a means of resolving personal conflict

[5] The institutional church had a resident minister and kindergartens, swimming pools, gyms, baths, clubs, libraries, dispensaries, clinics, open forums, classes, lectures, sewing and cooking schools, loan funds, penny savings banks, game rooms, soup kitchens, boardinghouse registries, employment services, and mutual benefit societies. Some of the institutional churches eventually developed hospitals and colleges. Temple University in Philadelphia, for example, is an outgrowth of a Baptist church.

[6] Davis (1959) hypothesizes that the traditional professions of the law, teaching, and the ministry were losing prestige to the business executive. Those who entered settlement work frequently had parents in the professions, parents who were either sympathetic to or were themselves abolitionists. The new social service seemed a perfect way to carry on the reform tradition of their families and at the same time to enter a new profession, which for women particularly, was open and promising. Woods and Kennedy (1922) assert that the outstanding achievement of the settlement movement substantiated, in no small means, women's claim to full acceptance in governmental affairs, an acceptance which might not have been achieved as readily through another field.

and putting into action the views of society to which they had been exposed in their college classrooms.[7]

While a great many young ministers and other socially conscious men eventually entered the settlement houses, of much greater importance to the movement was the influx of the young, highly educated women of that day. Seventy percent of the residents in the 250 most important houses were women (Woods & Kennedy, 1922). Jane Addams, Lillian Wald, Florence Kelley, Julia Lathrop, Alice Hamilton, Grace and Edith Abbott, Mary Simkhovich, Vida Scudder, and Jane Robbins were brilliant women with law and medical degrees, with M.A.'s and Ph.D.'s (Davis, 1959). These were the first generation of women for whom higher education became a reality. The women's

[7] There were, of course, a variety of motives bringing workers.

> All settlements are familiar with the sentimentalist caught by a shallow sympathy for and desire to help the poor, but who fails in fundamental democracy, humility and resource when brought face to face with normal people of an industrial neighborhood. Certain men and women are attracted by a supposedly ascetic flavor and undertake residence as a sort of moral scourging under which they hope to be unhappily happy. Closely related to this type is the missionary, the man or woman enamored of duty for duty's sake, and the charity-monger.
>
> A small number of men and women seek residence either to tide over an interim, or to find an agreeable place to stay, or to gain what they suppose will be a better social station. An occasional candidate labors under the delusion that he or she can in some way escape binding restrictions in another environment, but falls away after discovering that an industrial neighborhood is not in any sense a Bohemia, and that the very seriousness of experiments under way precludes the settlement from encouraging or tolerating a variety of irresponsible fancies.
>
> A certain number of men and women without consciousness of special vocation are attracted in the hope that actual contact with human life and need will discover them to themselves. An occasional person is received on this basis and allowed to test out his interests and powers in the widest and freest way. In their own self-education, settlement workers often apply the principle which governs so much of their class work, namely, that of allowing the individual to touch life at a sufficient number of different points to discover his mind (Woods & Kennedy, 1922, pp. 428–429).

To use Erikson's helpful term, for many the settlement house seemed to have served as the institution in which they could indulge in a "psycho-social moratorium." To view the settlement workers as neurotic, guilt-ridden do-gooders, as some do (Lasch, 1965), misses the point. As Lynd (1961) shows, the best of the settlement workers were radical reformers, with a definite social philosophy (Woods, 1906).

colleges had recently begun to grant degrees. The women who received them, often ardent feminists, often taught by socially conscious, ardent feminists, were determined not only to demonstrate that their intellectual productions were worthy, but they were impelled to justify their own existence by making themselves useful in the world (Linn, 1935).

Jane Addams, in her autobiography, *Twenty Years at Hull House,* tells how for several years after her graduation from college she travelled aimlessly, trying to decide upon a direction for her life. Through her travels, she became aware of the terrible poverty which existed, but she felt helpless about dealing with it.

> For two years in the midst of my distress over the poverty, which, thus suddenly driven into my consciousness, had become to me the "Weltschmerz", there was mingled a sense of futility, of misdirected energy, the belief that the pursuit of cultivation would not in the end bring either solace or relief. I gradually reached a conviction that the first generation of college women had taken their learning too quickly, had departed too suddenly from the active emotional life led by the grandmothers and great-grandmothers, that the contemporary education of young women had developed too exclusively the power of acquiring knowledge and of merely receiving impressions; that somewhere in the process of "being educated" they had lost that simple and almost automatic response to the human appeal, that old healthful reaction resulting in activity from the mere presence of suffering or helplessness (Addams, 1910, p. 71).

In 1888 she decided to establish a settlement house and visited Toynbee Hall for ideas. She felt she had found a mission for her life. In reviewing those years of indecision, years she had thought of as "preparation," she concluded:

> It was not until years afterward that I came upon Tolstoy's phrase "the snare of preparation" which he insists we spread before the feet of young people, hopelessly entangling them in a curious inactivity at the very period of life when they are longing to construct the world anew and to conform it to their own ideals (Addams, 1910, p. 88).

In a speech originally given in 1892, she further articulated the motives of the young settlement house worker. A better statement of the feelings and the problem of alienated youth can hardly be found.

This paper is an attempt to analyze the motives which underlie a movement based, not only upon conviction, but upon genuine emotion, wherever educated young people are seeking an outlet for that sentiment of universal brotherhood, which the best spirit of our times is forcing from an emotion into a motive. These young people accomplish little toward the solution of this social problem, and bear the brunt of being cultivated into unnourished, oversensitive lives. They have been shut off from the common labor by which they live which is a great source of moral and physical health. They feel a want of harmony between their theory and their lives, a lack of coordination between thought and action. I think it is hard for us to realize how seriously many of them are taking to the notion of human brotherhood, how eagerly they long to give tangible expression to the democratic ideal. . . .

We have in America a fast growing number of cultivated young people who have no recognized outlet for their active faculties. They hear constantly of the great social maladjustment, but no way is provided for them to change it, and their uselessness hangs about them heavily. Huxley declares that the sense of uselessness is the severest shock which the human system can sustain, and that if persistently sustained, it results in atrophy of function. These young people have had the advantages of college, of European travel, and of economic study, but they are sustaining this shock of inaction. . . . They tell their elders with all the bitterness of youth that if they expect success from them in business or politics or in whatever lines their ambition for them has run, they must let them consult all of humanity; that they must let them find out what the people want and how they want it. It is only the stronger young people, however, who formulate this. Many of them dissipate their energies in so-called enjoyment. Others not content with that, go on studying and go back to college for their second degrees; not that they are especially fond of study, but because they want something definite to do, and their powers have been trained in the direction of mental accumulation. Many are buried beneath this mental accumulation which lowered vitality and discontent. . . . This young life, so sincere in its emotion and good phrase and yet so undirected, seems to me as pitiful as the other great mass of destitute lives. One is supplementary to the other, and some method of communication can surely be devised. . . . Our young people feel nervously the need of putting theory into action, and respond quickly to the settlement form of activity (Addams, 1910, pp. 115–122).

The settlement house grew out of moral fervor and intellectual ideals, out of the need of the young educated person to find a useful place for himself, out of the complementary needs of the men, women, and children struggling to live in the massive urban slums created by an industrial might which produced both progress and poverty. In the settlement house, the two classes could meet and gain in fellowship because they were acting in a common purpose toward the satisfaction of mutual needs.

The fact that a predominant source of inspiration for the early settlement house workers came from the university gave the movement an intellectual bent which it retained in its emphasis on developing a scientific base for social reform. The broad intellectual character and the research orientation of this early movement in social work stands in marked contrast to the narrower emphasis on clinical method and psychoanalytic theory which later came to characterize the professional schools. In a real sense, the reforms accomplished by the settlement workers in the early 1900's, and even the marked changes of the 1930's, initiated by many who had been in the early settlements, were born in the seminar rooms and lecture halls of the universities.

the establishment of the first settlement houses

The first settlements were established in the late 1880's and the early 1890's in similar ways, many independently of each other. When

Stanton Coit returned from Toynbee Hall, he became an assistant to Felix Adler who had some ten years earlier founded the Ethical Culture Society, a group deeply involved in social and religious reform. Taking his inspiration from Toynbee Hall, within the year Coit located himself in a small tenement house on the Lower East Side of New York City. His initial reception by the neighborhood is quite amusing and worth recounting, not only as an anecdote, but because it gives something of a feeling of the times.

Coit at first intended to seek out an apartment in the worst tenement in the neighborhood where one tenth of all arrests for crime and one half of all arrests for gambling in the city of New York took place (Freeman, 1961). At the insistence of concerned friends he visited the local police station. When police officials could not offer even fair assurance for his physical safety, he decided to take a place in a somewhat quieter building nearby.

> The expressman called to move Dr. Coit's goods downtown protested at first that his client was in error concerning the address, and later was inclined to question his sanity. Neighbors were hardly less puzzled. A myth sprang up that he was a cast-off son of wealthy parents who had sought the East Side in the last descending stages of want. Popular sympathy was altogether with the supposed victim, and his family was hotly criticized for driving into such an environment anyone tenderly brought up. Only a dime novel plot seemed adequate to explain so unusual a situation as his presence in the district (Woods & Kenney, 1922, p. 42).

During the summer and fall, he cultivated the people in the neighborhood. He organized picnics for young people and later offered his apartment as a meeting place for a group of young men. From these beginnings came the concept of the club, and then the Neighborhood Guild, which eventually grew into the University Settlement.

The second settlement grew from the first. Dr. Jane E. Robbins and Jean Fine had worked with Coit for a while, but within a year the two women rented their own quarters nearby and began to organize clubs for girls. Several years earlier, under the impetus of Vida Scudder, a group of Smith College alumnae had gotten together to secure support for such a project. An association for the "support and control" of college settlements for women was organized with representation from Bryn Mawr, Vassar, and Wellesley. The project ripened none too soon, for the ward leader, "the notorious 'Silver Dollar' Smith," their heartless landlord, dispossessed them on the pretext that the traffic of the young girls of the neighborhood was wearing out the stairs in the apartment building. Coit had earlier started a campaign to obtain cleaner streets and it may be that the shrewd "Silver Dollar," quickly recognizing the settlement workers as potential enemies, acted to get rid of them (Woods & Kennedy, 1922).

At any rate, in the fall of 1889, a group of seven young women moved into a house on Rivington Street to start the College Settlement. Their first caller there was the local cop on the beat, who assumed the only reason a group of young women would rent a house on the Lower East Side was for "business" reasons. He offered not to interfere, provided the young women made an appropriate payoff (Davis, 1959). Undaunted, the women hung out a sign offering baths for five cents (no one came at first); they organized clubs for boys and girls, established a library, assisted at a Sunday school, took in a sick baby and nursed it back to health, and put up for the night a mother and her children who needed a temporary sanctuary from a husband in a drunken rage (Freeman, 1961). They made themselves useful in a friendly way, calling upon and receiving calls from their neighbors.

Lillian Wald, a graduate of Miss Cruttenden's *English-French Boarding and Day School for Young Ladies and Little Girls,* entered the school of nursing at New York Hospital. Wishing to make herself useful after graduating, she taught nursing to immigrant women in a Sabbath school whose purpose was to select candidates for nursing schools. Encountering the disorder and the misery of the neighborhood, she determined to find a place where she could be of greater assistance. With a friend she spent two months at the College Settlement, and then in 1893 the two women took an apartment on Jefferson Street, despite the anxieties of their parents.

The immigrant neighbors were ambivalent at first, concerned that the two were religious missionaries, but they were also pleased that "Americans" had come to live among them. The depression of 1893–1894 created even greater misery among the poor. Ministering to the sick, playing with the children, getting confirmation clothing for a little girl, sending an orphan to her mother's home in Rochester, ordering her nursing uniforms from a woman trying to support herself by sewing, interceding with public agencies, all established Miss Wald and her friend as persons who wanted to help. In a short time the neighbors came to tell their troubles, to seek advice, or just to talk.

Within two years, the project expanded so that the small apartment was no longer sufficient. The enterprise, now taking on the characteristics of a full-fledged settlement, was established on Henry Street as the Nurses' Settlement.[8] Here the visiting nurse service, with their characteristic uniforms and arm bands, was established. Their nursing skills gave them entry and safe passage everywhere and also gave the women access to the problems of the neighborhood. Public school nursing and a vast variety of public health efforts developed from the Henry Street Settlement. When Lillian Wald later sought public health legislation, she had a safe base of power in the neighborhood, and indeed in the city (Wald, 1915; Duffus, 1938).

The most famous of the settlements was undoubtedly Hull House, established in Chicago in 1889 by Jane Addams. After diligent search in the company of city missionaries, newspaper reporters, and officers of the compulsory education department, and with the advice of an ex-mayor of Chicago, she selected Hull House on Halstead Street as a suitable site for her settlement. Her description of the area is valuable for it not only gives a feeling of the neighborhood, but it also reminds us that some things have not changed very much.

> Halstead Street is thirty-two miles long, and one of the great thoroughfares of Chicago. . . . For six miles . . . the street is lined with shops of butchers and grocers, with dingy and gorgeous saloons, and pretentious establishments for the sale of ready-made clothing. Polk Street, running west from Halstead Street, grows rapidly more prosperous; running a mile east to State Street, it grows steadily worse, and crosses a network of vice on the corners of Clark Street and Fifth Avenue. Hull House once stood in the suburbs, but the city

---

[8] A few years after the establishment of the Nurses' Settlement, the official name was changed to the Henry Street Settlement. Legend has it that the athletic clubs were at a disadvantage in inter-settlement competition because at the height of battle, the opposition would unnerve them with the taunt, "Noices! Noices!" (Duffus, 1938).

has steadily grown up around it[9] and its site now has corners on three or four foreign colonies (Addams, 1910, pp. 97–98).

After describing the varied ethnic composition of the area, she goes on to say:

> The policy of the public authorities of never taking an initiative, and always waiting to be urged to do their duty, is obviously fatal in a neighborhood where there is little initiative among the citizens. The idea underlying our self-government breaks down in such a ward. The streets are inexpressibly dirty, the number of schools inadequate, sanitary legislation unenforced, the street lighting bad, the paving miserable and altogether lacking in the alleys and smaller streets, and the stables foul beyond description. Hundreds of houses are unconnected with the street sewer. The older and richer inhabitants seem anxious to move away as rapidly as they can afford it. They make room for the newly arrived immigrants who are densely ignorant of civic duties. This substitution of the older inhabitants is accomplished industrially also. . . . One of the most discouraging features about the present system of tenement houses is that many are owned by sordid and ignorant immigrants. The theory that wealth brings responsibility, that possession entails at length education and refinement, in these cases fails utterly. . . . Another thing that prevents better houses in Chicago is the tentative attitude of the real estate men. Many unsavory conditions are allowed to continue which would be regarded with horror if they were considered permanent. Meanwhile, the wretched conditions persist until at least two generations of children have been born or reared in them (Addams, 1910, pp. 98–100).

Like the other settlement workers, Jane Addams and Ellen Starr, her companion, were greeted with a certain amount of suspicion by the

---

[9] Elsewhere she described the house as having an undertaking establishment on one side and a saloon on the other, leading some wag to call the three "Knight, Death, and the Devil."

neighborhood. Jane Addams quotes a man who said their presence in the neighborhood was the strangest thing he had ever seen. The two women found they had an early ambassadress to the community in the person of a girl who came to live with them to do housework, but became an important worker in the first few years. The Hull House group came to their neighborhood with the articulated mission of sharing their cultural possessions with their new neighbors in order to establish the conditions for a fuller life in the area. One of the first activities was to start a reading party, in which a group of young women from the area met to listen and to discuss readings from George Eliot and from Hawthorne.

Another early activity was a kindergarten. The following anecdote suggests something of the problem of cultural difference and the attitude of the young workers toward their neighbors:

> One day at luncheon she gaily recited her futile attempt to impress temperance principles upon the mind of an Italian mother, to whom she had returned a small daughter of five sent to the kindergarten "in quite a horrid state of intoxication" from the wine-soaked bread upon which she had breakfasted. The mother, with the gentle courtesy of a South Italian, listened politely to her graphic portrayal of the untimely end awaiting so immature a wine bibber; but long before the lecture was finished, quite unconscious of the incongruity, she hospitably set forth her best wines, and when her baffled guest refused one after the other, she disappeared, only to quickly return with a small dark glass of whiskey, saying reassuringly, "See, I have brought you the true American drink." The recital ended in serio-comic despair, with the rueful statement that "the impression I probably made upon her darkened mind was that it is the American custom to breakfast children on bread soaked in whiskey instead of light Italian wine (Addams, 1910, pp. 102–103).

From the first, the desire to help was expressed in concrete personal service. Jane Addams and Ellen Starr washed newborn babies, prepared the dead for burial, nursed the sick, acted as midwives at the birth of an illegitimate baby, and took in a fifteen-year-old bride who was desperate to escape the nightly beatings administered by her husband. They became true neighbors, exchanging visits, sharing meals, attending weddings and christenings, becoming godparents, and participating in the life of the community by their sheer enjoyment of human contact. Just as the other settlement workers did, Jane Addams and Ellen Starr made a place for themselves in the neighborhood by giving of themselves.

Powdermaker's (1966) discussion of the anthropological technique of participant observation suggests to us that the early settlement workers shared with anthropologists intuitions about how to enter and become part of strange communities. The later professionals seem to have lost to their professionalism, as Jane Addams said so well, "that old healthful reaction resulting in activity from the mere presence of suffering or helplessness." They were not simply making people dependent on them. They were establishing a firm base in the community for later action. Perhaps there is a lesson here for the contemporary community mental health movement.

life in the settlement houses

While the quality of the settlement houses varied, life in the settlements at its best must have been an exciting experience spiced with vigorous intellectual interchange. At several of the houses opinion of all kinds was heard and tolerated and subjected to argument. In fact, the settlements were outstanding bastions of free speech in those days (Woods & Kennedy, 1922). The excitement was enhanced by the continual turnover of young residents, who came with a variety of purposes and from a variety of fields. There were young scientists and medical students, ministers and graduate students, wealthy dilettantes, ardent feminists, and social actionists of many different kinds. Journalists, novelists, and muckrakers came to the settlements seeking material. All were absorbed in common work and had a common cause. From this intellectual ferment came hundreds upon hundreds of books and articles, both scientific and popular in nature, and hundreds more of research studies concerning the social problems of the day. Woods and Kennedy (1911; 1922) list extensive bibliographies.

The residential quarters of the settlements were simple, but by no means austere, since they were usually large houses formerly owned by the well-to-do. At first, residents in a group would rent apartments nearby or in the same building, but these were usually uncomfortable. In the relatively small settlement buildings such as Hull House and Henry Street, living arrangements at first were much as in a family. Later rooms resembled college dormitories. The dining room frequently served as a common room, while a few of the houses had a residents' living room, with fireplace, piano, and a sociological library. The rooms at Hull House were well furnished and had paintings, photographs, and books.

Both male and female residents lived in the same building. The coeducational character of the settlements was the cause of some concern to the head workers, although it was considered desirable to have younger and older, men and women, and single and married people in the same center. A few settlements had accommodations for married couples and for families. However, few families remained in residence, primarily because they felt the immediate neighborhoods did not provide suitable environments for their children.

The residents tried to share the life of the neighborhood, but for some, differences in life style and in material wealth between them and their neighbors caused considerable personal conflict. The residents had feelings not terribly different from those experienced by some workers in anti-poverty programs who find themselves prospering, while the meaningful changes which can be observed are pitifully small compared with the magnitude of the problem. An example is found in the following excerpt:

> His family lived at the settlement of the Commons and he had a five months old baby. On the day that it was born a child was born in the family living across the street from the settlement. The two mothers had exchanged messages and afterward had become well acquainted, finding their motherhood a strong interest in common. When he and his wife noticed, however, that the other baby was not kept nearly so clean as their baby, they had to remind themselves that the mother across the street did all her own work and had a hard struggle to get on. Then it was difficult to get good milk in their neighborhood; even with

a refrigerator and other conveniences the milk spoiled, and when the mother across the way asked how they fed their baby and they replied that they used ———, she said, with a sigh, "yes, but that costs too much." It did cost. . . . Here at one blow was cut away all the common ground between them. How could they advise, how could they confer, how could they pretend to help the family across the way when the conditions under which they were living were so different, when they were not on the same economic basis at all? For his part, the matter had given him sleepless nights, his heart torn by the thought that their pretense of being helpful in the neighborhood was a mere sham, that until economic conditions were changed, they were utterly helpless (Richmond, 1961, p. 262).

In keeping with the democratic ideals of the settlements, most of the early houses were conducted on cooperative principles. In weekly meetings the residents decided details of cooperative housekeeping, house rules, and the nature of the work to be undertaken in the neighborhood. The members did much of their own work. While Jane Addams did take in a girl to help out, the girl became an integral part of the household, participating in the work of the settlement. Jane Addams frequently took her along when she addressed middle-class groups in order to have her respond to questions about life in the Hull House neighborhood. Although Jane Addams had two rooms for her own use, she insisted that her bath be shared by others. Lillian Wald and her companion did all their own work except for scrubbing and laundry. Residents took turns serving on the various committees responsible for the operation of the household.

Each person was encouraged to accept the challenge of developing and working up to his own highest standard. The basic responsibility for decisions and for implementation was left to individual workers. At Henry Street, each nurse was responsible for the management of her own patients and arranged her time according to her own best judgment. A family council was available to discuss problems and difficult situations, as well as issues of interest to the group (Duffus, 1938).

Most of the settlements had periodic meetings about the meaning of settlement work. The discussions led by the headworkers centered on broad questions of reform, problems of neighborhood organization, means of bringing culture to the people of the neighborhood, and interpretations of science, literature, philosophy, and religion in relation to the residents' personal outlooks. Invited speakers frequently came to discuss research or their observations of other communities and foreign countries.

The seminar was not the only medium of intellectual exchange. The dinner table was an important place for intellectual intercourse. Because meals were inexpensive, young intellectuals would come to the settlements to dine. Rube Borough, Ben Lindsey's coauthor, recalls that he and his friend, Carl Sandburg, frequently dined at Hull House in the early 1900's. Holden (1922), who was a settlement resident for a year or so, describes the scene:

> A favorite method of introduction is to get the stranger to take dinner with the residents. It will be a varied company. The women will probably be in the majority. There will be young women and middle-aged; there will be the well dressed attractive type and beside her the so-called "New England schoolmarm!" There will be long haired men in soft collars, whom the uninitiated will instantly suspect of socialism, as well as short haired men in business suits with conventional neck gear. There will be the inevitable buzz of conversation. Almost everyone will openly avow a genuine interest in what everyone else is doing and real importance will be attached to discussion of general topics of the day. There will be talking across the table, questionings, banterings, hasty opinions snapped and well considered opinions weighed. It is very possible that the visitor may feel himself talked to, cornered, even patronized by some one whom he does not know, asked to come again and almost forced to accept an invitation for the following week (Holden, 1922, pp. 35–36).

The intellectual caliber of the best of the houses can be judged (with some allowance for the adulation of authorized biographies) from the descriptions of some of the early residents.

> It is difficult to conceive of any attribute of Julia Lathrop that might be wished changed. She sparkled as did Florence

Kelley; their talk was a firework. . . . Mrs. Kelley was a
fighter; Miss Lathrop was a diplomat . . . when both were
at Hull House together, arguing some problem of correcting a social injustice, and disagreeing as they often did
on the best method of procedure, it is doubtful if any better
talk was to be heard anywhere. Prime Ministers of Europe,
philosophers of all doctrines, labor leaders and great capi-
talists and unpopular poets and popular novelists and
shabby exiles from half the kingdoms of the world visited
Hull House and dined there, and listened willingly . . .
and were glad to be there; and if they had only known it,
in the "house meetings" afterward, which only residents
attended, they would have heard more vivid discussions
still, sternly practical, yet still enlivened by the same
patient or impatient humor, as the case might be (Linn,
1935, pp. 140–141).

In recent years, historians and others interested in the development of ideas have given the settlement workers renewed recognition
both for intellectual and social accomplishments. Jane Addams' contribution to the development of the Chicago school of social science is
increasingly acknowledged. Indirect but important intellectual influences on Harry Stack Sullivan and John Dewey, for example, have
been attributed to Jane Addams and to Hull House (Lynd, 1961;
Sullivan, 1964; Lasch, 1965; 1967; Bernstein, 1967). As we shall see,
legislation regulating child labor and women's work, tenement laws,
sanitation codes, regulations promoting health and welfare, improvements in schools, the Juvenile Court movement, and similar reforms
developed directly or indirectly from the research and activities of
settlement workers. Still later, in the 1930's, much social and welfare
legislation was written, or influenced in its form and content, by
people who had been active in the earlier settlement house movement (Chambers, 1963).

The intellectual and research activities of the settlement workers
were among their most important contributions. William James said of
Jane Addams' first book, *Democracy and Social Ethics* (1902), "The
religion of democracy needs nothing so much as sympathetic interpretation to one another of the different classes of which society consists;
and you have made your contribution in a masterly manner."
Similarly the editor of the *San Francisco Bulletin* commented on how

Jane Addams' book had helped him to understand and to interpret to his readers the social and political conditions of the period.

As Davis (1959) summarized it, the settlement workers' research and their experiences put them in a position to know the problems firsthand, while their backgrounds enabled them to interpret the issues to the middle class and to political leaders and help effect sweeping social change through legislative action.

Professional activities were part of a full life and not separated from other aspects of living. The settlement workers intended to promote an intellectually and culturally rich democratic life among those they served and they wisely began by applying their principles to themselves. It is unfortunate that as the houses grew, a more authoritarian structure became necessary; but in the early days, by design, the way in which the workers treated each other generalized to the way in which they treated those whom they served in the neighborhoods. While there is a distinct danger in oversentimentalizing the past, one cannot help but feel more than a touch of envy of those who had the privilege of sharing in the fellowship of the early settlement houses.

how the settlements were financed

Consideration of the financial arrangements of the settlements is necessary, for any group bent on social reform needs financial independence. The settlement workers soon learned that "he who pays the piper calls the tune."

Most of the earliest houses were founded and financed by a group of unsalaried residents who rented their own quarters. Later, when groups moved into houses, the residents paid for their room and board. While many worked full time in the settlement, others had jobs which gave them time for settlement work. The financial situation changed as the backgrounds of the residents changed. Not all who came later had the independent income of a Jane Addams or a Lillian Wald. In the absence of independent incomes, fellowships for young students and salaries for full-time residents and other employees became necessary.

The level of salaries presented a set of problems. The residents' principles demanded that secretaries, domestics, janitors, and handymen receive living wages, but the settlements' finances often led to underpaid employees. Similarly, the salaries of the residents themselves were a problem. Too little money led to anxiety about illness and dependence in old age, while higher wages created guilt feelings in the workers. There was a tendency to set salary scales in accordance with what educators received.

Once the settlements entered the fund raising business, they found that the flow of funds sometimes depended on action, or inaction, which might compromise the independence and the ideals of the settlements. There are three major sources of funds for enterprises such as settlements: the government; private philanthropy; and subscriptions, memberships, and fees for settlement activities. Settlement workers in the early days rejected government (municipal) support, not only because they frequently were at odds with city governments but also because they experimented with a variety of services they hoped government facilities would adopt later (e.g., kindergartens, visiting teachers, probation officers). Settlement leaders felt their freedom to innovate and experiment would be seriously compromised if they worked within the framework of governmental agencies.

This was before the days of massive federal support of social welfare projects, but experience today suggests the settlement workers hit upon an important truth. No agency of government can afford to finance its critics, nor can it legitimately finance revolutionaries. The experience of Mobilization for Youth in New York and recent legislative efforts to limit activities of the Office of Economic Opportunity programs speak loud and clear. While government might be benevolent, and in its benevolence promote important changes, there is probably a narrow limit to the changes government can tolerate at any point in time.

Some of the settlement houses raised a substantial portion of their funds from the neighborhoods they served but in most of the houses neighborhood support amounted to about 10 percent of the budgets. In a few instances all of the necessary funds were raised from within the neighborhoods and no other outside source of support was necessary or desired. It was the opinion of some that all support should be raised from the neighborhoods, but that proved difficult. The settlements served poor people who did not have the money to contribute. In some instances, even where some money was raised from the immediate area, the bulk of subscriptions came from "uptown" members. Some of the settlements with larger budgets tended to disregard the monies which could be raised from neighborhoods because they felt it was too difficult, or too unimportant to be worthy of much effort (Woods & Kennedy, 1922; Holden, 1922).

Probably the two most important sources of funds were wealthy individuals and organizations such as the Junior League. Funds from large donors were exceedingly important for building and developing endowments. However, these funds were not without their problems. For one, the funds were often given for specific purposes and were not available for the general purposes of the settlements (Holden, 1922). For another, a settlement would become dependent upon the good will of one or a few wealthy patrons. If the patron became displeased, a settlement would be faced with a sudden withdrawal of funds, and Woods and Kennedy (1922) point out that almost all of the active settlements, at one time or another, took stands on controversial issues which cost them patronage.

High-spirited individuals such as Jane Addams and Lillian Wald did not back away from controversy, even though their activities cost them support. In 1899, a dozen colored women, delegates to a congress held in Chicago, were invited to lunch at Hull House. As a consequence, southern editors "uninvited" Jane Addams to speak in the South, and speaking was an important source of income for her. In another instance, she defended a young man falsely arrested as an anarchist after the assassination of President McKinley. Her support of the young man cost her the patronage of a Chicago socialite and won her the castigation of several socially prominent ministers. Her pacifist and anti-war stands lost her considerable support later on (Linn, 1935). Lillian Wald, very active in anti-war organizations, also suffered a loss of financial support because of her activities (Duffus, 1938). Later, after the war, when the political climate was anti-Red and the settlements were considered hotbeds of radicalism, they had great difficulty in raising money for anything more than fresh air camps or Americanization classes to teach English to immigrants (Holden, 1922).

Sometimes proffered funds were in the nature of a bribe. Hull House once turned down a gift of $50,000 which was dependent upon the residents ceasing agitation for a factory law in Illinois. It is a measure of the stature of Jane Addams that she did not congratulate herself for having turned down the bribe, but rather felt mortified that someone had even thought to offer it to her.

The means through which wealthy patrons earned their money caused other problems for the settlements. There was a great deal of discussion about "tainted money," an issue which arose when Jane Addams turned down a contribution of $20,000 for a building for the Jane Club, a cooperative apartment dwelling for working girls, because the donor was notorious for underpaying his female employees (Addams, 1910; Linn, 1935). As Jane Addams pointed out so clearly, the issues were often confused, but the fact that the issues arose at all suggests the settlements, at least in their earlier days, were determined to maintain their independence and their freedom to question any aspect of society including "that dubious area wherein wealth is accumulated."

Wealthy patrons who were morally committed and who had no fear of consequences were vitally important to the work of the major settlements. Jane Addams' biographer provides a brief sketch of Mrs. Joseph T. Bowen, who for many years was closely involved with Hull House and with the development of the Juvenile Court in Chicago (see Chapter 8). Mrs. Bowen, a wealthy aristocrat, was never a resident, but she joined the Hull House Women's Club, soon becoming president, an office she held for seventeen years. As president, as organizer of the Juvenile Protective Association, and as president of the Chicago Juvenile Court Committee, she was actively engaged in social reform. She could bring intimate knowledge to her work as trustee and treasurer of the Hull House Association, as could many of the settlement board members who frequently carried several responsibilities within a settlement.

The attitudes of patrons such as Mrs. Bowen can be gleaned from this description of her by Jane Addams' biographer.

> Rooted in conservatism, a patriot of the old school, proud of her long record of "Black Republicanism", Mrs. Bowen surveyed some of the activities, a few of the residents, and many of the visitors to Hull House with a severe though humorous eye. She liked things the way she liked them, and eccentric manifestations of radicalism she never liked; nor did she ever join the Women's International League for Peace. But she no more dreamed of

forcible interference with the opinions of other people than she dreamed of the possibility that any one might successfully interfere with her own opinions, and took the same pride in the hospitality of Hull House to every shade of political expression that she took in her own hospitality to every sort of guest. To oddity of all sorts she opposed merely a kind of queenly acceptance. Jane Addams herself, in Mrs. Bowen's view, might think strangely, but she could never do wrong, any more than Mrs. Bowen herself could be mean; both conceptions were impossible. For four decades, Mrs. Bowen has retained a sense of feudality in connection with Hull House, a consciousness that noblesse oblige. She has laughed at herself, laughed at what she has regarded as centrifugal, laughed at everything except service and fineness; those two are the articles of her creed (Linn, 1935, pp. 143–144).

In order that policies be kept responsive to the needs of the neighborhood, it was necessary to keep board members in close touch with the settlements' work. Aristocrats such as Mrs. Bowen were invaluable, and an attempt was made to have board members take on volunteer work and club leadership. Past presidents were encouraged to return as board members. The active engagement of the board with the resident staff and with the people of the neighborhood was encouraged in order to keep boards alert to local needs.

Actually, there seem to have been few instances in which there was neighborhood representation on boards; generally it was found difficult to interest workingmen in participating, and in view of the necessity that the board accept financial responsibility, it was not useful to have poor people represented.

The poor were represented on house councils, which were often delegated some degree of power by the board (one group had the authority to impeach the headworker, for example). They were also represented on the boards of financial associations, groups consisting of those who contributed to the settlement, or were members by virtue of the fees they paid (Woods & Kennedy, 1922).

Nonetheless, it was difficult to guarantee that the policy-making boards would be responsive to the needs of the neighborhood. Not all board members were as tolerant and open as Mrs. Bowen. Woods and Kennedy (1922) and Holden (1922) allude to the various problems which developed around boards. Holden felt that the chief qualification for many board members was the money they were able to contribute, a fact which did not dampen their enthusiasm, but which probably meant they would not have the knowledge and experience of the residents.

The problem of control by boards in later years is presented in a light which makes some of the settlements seem rather pathetic. Holden (1922) reprinted a "settlement catechism" written by Mary Kingsbury Simkhovitch about 1912. It sets forth a view of the settlement in somewhat simplistic terms. With respect to the board, the catechism states:

> If the settlement is a family, what is the Settlement's Committee or Board of Managers?
>
> Such boards are friends of the family who help it to carry on its neighborhood enterprises and give it counsel. Such a board may properly refuse to give support to any enterprise in which it does not believe or may encourage by financial help that in which it does believe.
>
> Is such a board necessary?
>
> It or something similar is necessary unless the Settlement family is entirely self-sustaining, and this rarely is the case (Holden, 1922, p. 192).

The original democratic organization gave way to an authoritarian structure as the settlements' financial needs grew. Was the loss of self-determination entirely necessary? Woods and Kennedy (1922) argue that the best-financed settlements tended to be the least active and the most complacent. The more politically active settlements were characterized by continual financial struggles. However, even though settlements bold in their approach tended to lose some short-run support, over the long haul the more outspoken and active of the settlements found they could depend upon admiring followers to see them through financial stresses.

Leadership of the settlements was also an important consideration. A strong leader with a moral commitment to settlement ideals could not conscientiously do anything other than attempt to live up to his personal ideals. The later generations of settlement leaders, coming as they did from professional schools and having the careerist rather than the crusader viewpoint, were, understandably, less concerned with independence. They had programs, payrolls, and buildings to concern them, inheritances of the successes of the previous generation of settlement workers.

Moreover, professionalism in social work also influenced the new group coming to the settlement houses in the 1920's and the 1930's (See Chapter 10). As graduates of professional schools with training in scientific casework and scientific group work, they were no longer concerned with social reform, particularly in the conservative 1920's. Sons and daughters of immigrants who became settlement workers and who had been brought up in the slums were not interested in living in the slums, nor in remaining there after hours. Settlement work became a job, and there was a conscious attempt to give the job a professional status. The enthusiasm and the commitment of the earlier era was no longer there in the same degree among the later workers (Davis, 1959). In part, the settlement house movement fell victim to its own success.

the concept of community organization

Stanton Coit, the man who established the first settlement in the United States, came to the settlement concept with a plan. He intended to help a neighborhood become organized for its own development:

> The first step in social reform, if my psychology be correct, must be the conscious organization of the intellectual and moral life of the people for the total improvement of the human lot. . . . Because of the lack of it, our ideals and schemes are cold, abstract, bloodless things, or at best, are impotent. . . . If this first step, the organization of the masses mentally and morally, were taken, the second step, the enlightenment of the people in social principles, could be easily made, and then the realization of the just state would not be remote, nor would it be brought in with violence. Now such a general organization of the life of the people, and such a general civic instruction, are the special field of action which the Neighborhood Guild would presume to assign to itself (Coit, 1891, pp. 4–5).

The Neighborhood Guild was guided by definite concepts concerning the nature of urban industrial life. Recognizing the tendency for the authority of the family to decline, and recognizing the tendency for ties between people to become role specific rather than diffused, Coit saw the guild as an extension of the family concept in which members banded together to pursue many goals. He specifically decried the tendency of modern-day groups to be formed for single purposes, noting that such single-purpose association tended to overvalue the specific function and did not encourage people to know each other in more than a single dimension. The Neighborhood Guild, by drawing people together in an alliance to promote and to carry out "all the reforms—domestic, industrial, educational, provident, or recreative— which the social ideal demands," would bring greater advantage. "The supreme aim which it constantly keeps in view is the completest efficiency of each individual, as a worker for the community, in morals, manners, workmanship, civic virtues and intellectual power, and the fullest possible attainment of social and industrial advantages" (Coit, 1891, p. 11).

The guild was not limited solely "to the rescue of those who have already fallen into vice, crime or pauperism." It would also direct itself toward the stable working class, for Coit saw himself engaged not only in preventive work, but in efforts to realize the highest ideals of the culture. "The way to save and prevent is often by educating the intellect, and cultivating the taste of the person in danger or already fallen; and, again, the superior development of one member of a family or of a circle of friends may prove the social salvation of all the rest" (Coit, 1891, pp. 11–12).

Coit recognized the numbers problem. The concept of mutual assistance and self-help was built in because he recognized that while it was possible for a small group to care for most of its own needs, it was impossible for any single association to serve everyone. He envisioned guilds which would propagate themselves through members organizing new groups in adjacent areas. Coit saw that only the force of self-help could begin to approach the magnitude of the problem. "If we consider the vast amount of personal attention and time needed, to understand and deal effectively with the case of any one man or family that has fallen into vice, crime or pauperism, we shall see the impossibility of coping with even these evils alone, unless the helpers be both many and constantly at hand" (Coit, 1891, p. 19).

However, Coit also pointed out that organized self-help did not exist: it arose spontaneously at a point of need. Neighbors know almost immediately when a family is in difficulty, and they understand the nature of the difficulty. Where an outsider comes necessarily as an inquisitor, a neighbor can know without prying. Neighbors do help each other in time of troubles; not only does the help take a concrete form but it is easier to accept from someone in similar circumstances. One does not become "a case." The giver of assistance and the receiver can identify with each other as having common needs. Coit comments: "It is terrible when men draw together only in suffering; whereas those who have laughed and thought together, and joined in ideal aims, can so enter into one another's sorrow as to steal much of its bitterness away" (Coit, 1891, p. 27).

the club: unit of organization

Within the settlements, the unit of organization was the club. The club usually consisted of a group of eight to twenty members but some grew as large as seventy. The members of the club organized themselves formally and remained together for years, the club serving as the reference group for the members. Each club had a leader who was not a member but who served as a guide and a counselor for the group. Following the principles of democratic organization, members elected their own officers, organized according to some set of rules, and conducted their business by parliamentary procedure. The club provided a laboratory for learning democratic process. The groups developed their own projects, decided upon their own entertainment, organized for their own education, and in some instances helped in political and social action.[10] While there were many clubs for younger children and for young adults, the club concept extended to include

[10] "When in 1902 New York's Reform Mayor Seth Low was running against Tammany, the American Hero Club (Henry Street's first club), made up of boys who had at first been disposed to throw decaying vegetables at the nurses under the impression they were missionaries, then had been won over to enthusiastic and lasting approval when they discovered they were friends, threw all their energies in the Low campaign and scattered campaign literature left and right" (Duffus, 1938, p. 87).

other people as well. Clubs were established which brought together
people with common concerns, but within the settlement clubs of
differing age, sex, and marital composition met together, and worked
and planned some activities cooperatively.

Holden (1922), who was a settlement house resident, describes
how a club was developed:

A certain group of boys averaging about fifteen or sixteen
years got the reputation of being "the toughest bunch on
the block!" They used to stand around drug stores and
side doors of saloons smoking very cheap cigarettes and cat-
calling at the girls who passed by. They had a scorn for the
conventional type of hats and affected big caps pulled over
their ears at curious angles. They had a peculiar way of
spitting out of the corners of their mouths. They punctuated
their sentences with words like Jesus and damn and hell,
and others not so nice in their original meaning. They spent
their evenings provoking trouble and hunting for excitement. One night they visited the neighborhood dance in
progress at a settlement (Admission 5 cents). Two of them
were kicked out for refusing to take off their caps, another
was evicted for a rough house that ended in breaking a
chair, a fourth was put out for using profane language.
Three remained. They were engaged in conversation by a
very large man they later learned had been a famous foot-
ball player at Princeton. They were interested in the
gymnasium equipment. The idea came to them that basketball could be played by boys who didn't go to high school.
They asked if they could play. They were told that if they
formed a club and had a director that they could play.
They asked the big man to be their director and said they
would get the rest of their "bunch." But the rest of the
bunch resentful over having been put out, refused to come
in. They asked the big man if he would come and talk to
the others. He did. He spent an evening with them. Where
they went he went also, but they noticed that he didn't cat-
call after girls and that he didn't wear a cap.

They came to the settlement house again and asked
him to spend another evening with them. The big man said

he didn't much enjoy dancing on cellar doors and proposed that they should go to a show. Two of them hadn't any money and asked him to wait while they "swiped a nickel off the soda and candy man at the corner." He said he'd lend them the money. They said that would be all right that "they'd swipe it later." They noticed that he took off his hat when he went into the movie house. They asked if they couldn't form a club and play basketball. He helped them start their club (Holden, 1922, pp. 67–69).

The section goes on to describe other ways in which the club leader helped the boys, getting them gym shoes, and helping them to earn money for club dues. Holden describes the ways in which the group began to identify with him. Once the club was organized, it became a part of the settlement itself, engaging in a variety of activities.

Women's and girls' clubs followed the same general pattern. If anything, some of the settlement workers felt these were even more successful because they had more leadership available. Details of how the clubs were organized and the varied purposes they served may be found in Addams (1910), in Wald (1915), and in Woods and Kennedy (1922). Unfortunately for our purposes, Woods and Kennedy (1922), the single most complete source describing the nature of settlement houses in the years before World War I, makes no mention of any formal studies of the effectiveness of the various clubs in promoting the development of youth or in preventing delinquency. However, Lillian Wald asserts that: "Although in the twenty-one years of the organized life of the settlement no girl or young woman identified with us has 'gone wrong" in the usual understanding of that term, we have been so little conscious of working definitely for this end that my attention was drawn to the fact only when a woman distinguished for her work among girls made the statement that never in the Night Court or institutions for delinquents had she found a girl who had 'belonged' to our settlement" (Wald, 1914, p. 174). Wald goes on to state that club members believed in the effectiveness of the control of the club as a means of preventing delinquencies among boys.

It is certainly true that many of the children, and even the older people of the neighborhoods, simply would not have been exposed to the educational, recreational, and cultural activities had the settlement not existed. By its consideration of contemporary problems, by athletics, classes, dramatics, and trips to the country, the settlements brought something to the neighborhood which otherwise would have been unavailable. Perhaps it is true that they reached only those who were able to take advantage of what they offered, but who can measure the significance of the settlement bridge to the thousands upon thousands who used it to pass from the ghettos and the slums into the larger society?

the settlements and education

The settlement movement attempted to educate both the larger society and the poor in the neighborhoods it served. Settlement workers believed that change would come about when people knew the facts and they eventually did achieve changes by educating people to the facts, facts they revealed through their own research. But their hypothesis, that social evils existed and persisted because of ignorance, needed considerable modification and qualification.

Contact with schools and homes showed the settlement workers they were in for an uphill battle, if they were to promote public education as a means of improving the lives of their neighbors. Many of their neighbors had neither interest nor faith in education. Some of the older immigrant families saw the schools, with their emphasis on Americanization, as a means of stealing away their children's loyalties (Woods, 1898). Many of the families needed their children to help in earning a living, and kept them out of school to work even when it was illegal to do so. Many of the parents took most if not all of the earnings of their children and expected to continue to do so. It was a tradition in some of the immigrant families that the children be brought up to believe it was their duty to care for their parents when their parents became too old to work. The schools' efforts to make the children independent were viewed as extremely threatening. It took great effort and great patience to change some of these attitudes (Lasch, 1965).

The schools themselves left much to be desired. Educators tended to view the foreigners who could not speak the language as ignorant and unteachable. The school system generally was dominated by ward politics (Cremin, 1964). "Schools in tenement neighborhoods showed the most serious fire risks, the most antiquated and insanitary quarters, the largest number of pupils to a class, and the least efficient teaching" (Woods & Kennedy, 1922, p. 275).

Settlement residents almost immediately became involved with school administration through campaigns to "keep the schools out of politics," as part of municipal reform, and through participation on central school boards and local committees of school trustees.[11] Jane Addams reported on her experiences with the Chicago School Board in *Hull House* (Addams, 1910).

Figures showing the prevalence of underfed children led to the development of penny lunch programs within the settlements. These programs, picked up by the Board of Education later, resulted in school lunch programs and provisions for mid-morning and mid-afternoon snacks for all children. Open air schools and classes as a means of treating tuberculosis were established on an experimental basis in a number of settlements and later adopted by the public schools.

Settlements were instrumental in starting the visiting teacher service, which we will discuss in Chapter 6. School nursing was established as an outgrowth of the visiting nurse service which was centered in the Henry Street Settlement. Other more direct educational innovations were also stimulated by the settlements. Many had kindergartens, and settlement workers used their influence among people in the neighborhood to stimulate a demand that the public schools provide the service. College extension classes, held in the settlements, played a part in starting a demand for public evening high schools. Classes for the handicapped and the mentally retarded were supported by the efforts of settlement residents. Their efforts were important in helping the public school accept such special needs within its own area of responsibility. While other groups originated the concept of teaching

[11] In relation to the current fight in New York City and elsewhere for local control of the schools, it would be of interest to explore school organization in this earlier period. Woods and Kennedy write: "A committee of these [local school] trustees had power to appoint and remove teachers and janitors, to contract for supplies, and to engage buildings. Such power was, however, so much abused that settlements took an active part in securing a law which relieved local school boards of the largest part of their administrative work. Many residents continued to serve on the reconstituted advisory groups" (1922, p. 276).

handwork and homemaking in the schools, the settlements pioneered in gaining acceptance for curricular change. They introduced such programs into the summer vacation schools they operated, and then pressed for their adoption in the regular curriculum.

Eventually several settlements were established by schoolteachers for schoolteachers, and one of these, on the Lower East Side, was supported by Julia Richman, one of the first female school executives in New York. That settlement became a center for conferences on school and community relations, and was highly influential among public school teachers (Woods & Kennedy, 1922).

Thousands of adults and children made full use of the extensive educational and recreational programs of the settlements (Addams, 1910; Woods & Kennedy, 1922; Lasch, 1965). The settlement workers also encouraged the children, developed their talents, and supported their efforts to get their parents to make the sacrifices necessary for further education. Families unable or unwilling to provide for their own children were helped by the resources of the settlements and the workers.

Not only did the settlements provide libraries, but the libraries and living rooms were used as places to study where residents helped with homework and organized small groups for remedial study. The settlements were there and available; the residents were there and accessible as models for the children who wanted to become educated Americans. The profound effect of the settlements cannot be measured, but it certainly cannot be questioned, and undoubtedly it must be respected.

the settlements, social action, and political involvement

Before beginning this study, we believed the settlement houses were glorified community centers which also provided some social services, that term being used in its contemporary, professional sense. In point of fact, of some 321 settlement houses established before 1910, about 80 percent were engaged solely in educational and recreational activities, while only 3 percent of the settlements were heavily involved in social and political action. Many of the settlements, about 16 percent, did engage in research and investigations of local conditions which had relevance for social action. Those settlements engaged in political activity and in socially relevant investigation were almost exclusively located in big cities, in areas where recent, Eastern European immigrants predominated. They were largely independent or university affiliated; rarely did they have institutional affiliations with churches, and most of their funds came from private sources.

These data, compiled from the Woods and Kennedy *Handbook of Settlements* (1911) by Levine and Levine (1967),[12] are a tribute to the power and the intellectual character of the early settlement movement. A handful of settlements with strong leadership and support from each other had the determination to forge tools of social research and of political action. In so doing, they improved in substantial ways the life conditions of people throughout the country. The story of the political and social action of the early settlements is worth recounting because these early settlements provide a model for contemporary community-oriented practice. There are also important lessons about what forms of social and political action are effective for the professional mental health worker to attempt.

clean streets and garbage

Stanton Coit lived on Forsyth Street for less than a year before he tried to organize a campaign for clean streets. Dirty, dimly lit streets served as storage places for trucks; dark, dirty halls and stairways and unlocked hallway doors and cellars were invitations to crime. Slimy and crowded sidewalks, the only playgrounds for children, aroused anger in the settlement workers who *lived in these conditions*. More articulate than the typical slum dweller, they complained loud and long to municipal officials, to newspaper reporters, and to influential friends. They got some action, but the amount of action was small in relation to their effort and in relation to their need. What they discovered was that municipal officials felt they could safely leave slum districts for

[12] This paper by David and Zachary Levine received a second place in the annual Hamden, Connecticut, Science Fair, April, 1967.

the last when improvements were considered because there was no aroused public complaining of the poor conditions.

In various ways, the settlements worked toward arousing neighborhood interest in improvements in the area. Club members formed associations which assumed responsibility for street cleaning. Some settlements established brigades of children to help in this work. The job was not easy. One of the reasons the immigrants did not complain was because their sanitary standards had always been low. Coming from villages where personal uncleanliness was neither offensive nor a danger to public health, the newcomers did not know how to use sanitary facilities, and would deposit waste in places where it did not belong, or just throw it out windows. (It was not yet called "air mailing!") Through pleading, persuasion, protests, and complaints to the police, encouraging them to enforce what laws there were, residents of the settlements got some action.

However, keeping a neighborhood clean is partly a function of the garbage collection and disposal services. At that time contracts for garbage collection were farmed out as political plums, and service was careless and irregular. At Hull House, after the Women's Club had reported over a thousand instances of inadequate service, and after Jane Addams lost out on a bid to become the local garbage contractor, she was appointed garbage inspector. She saw to it that the contractors did their duty. While vigorous activity (keeping charts and records, following garbage wagons to the dumps, arguing with the contractor, having landlords arrested, and complaining to City Hall) helped to clean up the neighborhood, Jane Addams became convinced that for permanent change it would be necessary to actively oppose the local political boss.[13]

13 Male residents were of critical importance in political action and some like Raymond Robins, a resident of Chicago Commons, were acknowledged past masters of ward politics (Davis, 1959). Women had not yet won the vote and were not well accepted in politics as the following letter addressed to Jane Addams will attest:

No man can love a woman who takes her place among men as you do. . . . And now for a little advice to help you defeat the good man you have so often tried to do without success of course, I can speak very plain to you, as your highest ambition is to be recognized as capable of doing a man's work. . . . Did it ever occur to you while on a tour of inspection, through alleyways old barns and such places where low depraved men with criminal records may be found (such a place a virtuous woman would be afraid to go.) You might for a

We shall return to the lessons which were derived from the several political campaigns in local politics, but for the moment it is important to sketch in some of the other accomplishments of the settlements in areas related to sanitation and housing and education. Residents were at the forefront of efforts to achieve improvements in the disposal of stockyard refuse to get rid of the local stench; to replace a municipal garbage dump with an incinerator; to obtain public baths in neighborhoods where tenements did not have running water or adequate facilities; and to obtain improvement in the schools.

While there were other groups seeking housing reforms, the settlement residents lived in tenement environments, intimately in touch with the problems and the people. They were able to do the necessary research to show the effects of existing conditions on the health and welfare of men, women, and children, upon standards of homemaking, child care, and sexual morality, and upon family structure. It was the settlement residents who in many cases documented the problems and provided the basis for corrective legislation. The laws were not ends in themselves, for the residents learned that vigilance in the enforcement of the laws was a necessary element in obtaining change. They found that enforcement really depended upon the community because neighbors "conspired together" to secure and to maintain standards.

The details of these fights are not important for our immediate purposes. What is important is that the efforts at social reform were carried through on the basis of the findings of participant observation and survey research, that each step of the research led to a broadened view of the problems of the neighborhood, and that the procedure represented a method for the empirical study of the social organization of communities. In effect, each effort at intervention could be characterized as an experiment in nature, designed to test an hypothesis concerning the social causes of observable phenomena, and each failure of an attempt at intervention led to a reformulation of the hypothesis of causation. Thus the settlement house workers developed a basis for

---

small sum induce one of such men to sell you his pecker and balls. It would not be much loss to him, and will be your only chance to prove yourself a man. You could then go before a board of examiners chosen from the 19th ward prove yourself capable of filling a man's place, You could then have the privelage of casting a vote, and should that bold bad Johnny Powers challenge you you could produce your pecker cast your vote, and probably defeat him (Lasch, 1965, p. XXI).

arriving at an understanding of the community and of how people lived in the community.

The efforts at intervention, as we have seen, first led the settlement workers into conflict with the local ward boss. In most instances, they found they really did not have the strength or the know-how for effective opposition. In some instances, the ward leader's opposition was sufficient to cause the settlement to close or to move. In fact, he was a master of the game of becoming important by providing direct assistance to people. Even the most corrupt of bosses served important and socially beneficial functions in their neighborhoods.

That political bosses and settlement workers saw themselves as rivals is easy to understand. The following passages, quoting George W. Plunkitt of Tammany Hall, show that their methods of reaching people were highly similar.[14]

> There's only one way to hold a district; you must study human nature and act accordin'. You can't study human nature in books. Books is a hindrance more than anything else. If you have been to college, so much the worse for you. You'll have to unlearn all you learned before you can get right down to human nature, and unlearnin' takes a lot of time. Some men can never forget what they learned at college. Such men may get to be district leaders by a fluke, but they never last.
>
> To learn real human nature you have to go among the people, see them and be seen. I know every man, woman and child in the Fifteenth District, except them that's been born this summer—and I know some of them too. I know what they like and what they don't like, what they are strong at and what they are weak in, and I reach them by approachin' at the right side.
>
> For instance, here's how I gather in the young men. I hear of a young feller that's proud of his voice, that he can sing fine. I ask him to come around to Washington Hall and join our Glee Club. He comes and sings, and he's a follower of Plunkitt for life. Another young feller gains a a reputation as a baseball player in a vacant lot. I bring

[14] See Woods (1898) and Lasch (1965) for similar descriptions of ward bosses in Boston and in Chicago.

him into our baseball club. That fixes him. You'll find him workin' for my ticket at the polls next election day. Then there's the feller that likes rowin' on the river, the young feller that makes a name as a waltzer on his block, the young feller that's handy with his dukes—I rope them all in by givin' them opportunities to show themselves off. I don't trouble them with political arguments. I just study human nature and act accordin'.

But you may say this game won't work with the high-toned fellers, the fellers that go through college and then join the Citizens' Union. Of course it wouldn't work. I have a special treatment for them. I ain't like the patent medicine man that gives the same medicine for all diseases. The Citizens' Union kind of a young man! I love him! He's the daintiest morsel of the lot, and he don't often escape me. . . .

I tell you frankly, though, how I have captured some of the Citizens' Union's young men. I have a plan that never fails. I watch the City Record to see when there's a civil service examination for good things. Then I take my young cit in hand, tell him all about the good things and get him worked up till he goes and takes an examination. I don't bother about him any more. It's a cinch that he comes back to me in a few days and asks to join Tammany Hall. Come over to Washington Hall some night and I'll show you a list of names on our rolls marked "C.S." which means, "bucked up against civil service. . . ."

What tells in holdin' your grip on your district is to go right down among the poor families and help them in the different ways they need help. I've got a regular system for this. If there's a fire in Ninth, Tenth, or Eleventh Avenue, for example, any hour of the day or night, I'm usually there with some of my election district captains as soon as the fire engines. If a family is burned out I don't ask whether they are Republicans or Democrats, and I don't refer them to the Charity Organization Society, which would investigate their case in a month or two and decide they were worthy of help about the time they are dead from starvation. I just get quarters for them, buy clothes for them if their clothes were burned up, and fix them up till they get things runnin' again. It's philanthropy, but it's politics, too—mighty good politics. Who can tell how many votes one of these fires bring me? The poor are the most grateful people in the world, and, let me tell you, they have more friends in their neighborhoods than the rich have in theirs.

If there's a family in my district in want I know it before the charitable societies do, and me and my men are first on the ground. I have a special corps to look up such cases. The consequence is that the poor look up to George W. Plunkitt as a father, come to him in trouble—and don't forget him on election day.

Another thing, I can always get a job for a deservin' man. I make it a point to keep on the track of jobs, and it seldom happens that I don't have a few up my sleeve ready for use. I know every big employer in the district and in the whole city, for that matter, and they ain't in the habit of sayin' no to me when I ask them for a job.

And the children—the little roses of the district! Do I forget them? Oh no! They know me, every one of them, and they know that a sight of Uncle George and candy means the same thing. Some of them are the best kind of vote-getters. I'll tell you a case. Last year a little Eleventh Avenue rosebud whose father is a Republican, caught hold of his whiskers on election day and said she wouldn't let go till he'd promise to vote for me. And she didn't (Riordan, 1905, pp. 46–53).

Settlement workers engaged in local politics to different degrees. The political leader in Robert Woods's district was apparently honest and benevolent. Woods found he could cooperate with him in many projects. In other areas, settlement workers ran for local office, oftentimes unsuccessfully. In some instances, settlement workers found it was not good to run for local office because they thus closed off important avenues of advancement for young neighborhood men. Some settlement workers felt that it was more effective not to run campaigns themselves, but to try to educate the local populace to demand more of the political boss. When the bosses could be shown that neighborhood improvement was in their interest, they would fight for and obtain improvements the settlement workers wanted. Often the settlement workers actively supported reform candidates, or good men regardless of party (Woods, 1898; Woods & Kennedy, 1922; Davis, 1959; Lasch, 1965).

Jane Addams' experience at Hull House with the local political leader is important to relate since we can already hear some in the contemporary community mental health movement argue that mental health workers and behavioral scientists must enter politics in order to achieve social change. There is a body of experience which suggests that such a view should be examined with great care.

Over a period of years, Hull House residents had clashed with the local ward leader on a number of issues. We have already discussed the problem of garbage. There were other areas in which a local boss was obstructive. For example, although Hull House maintained what was tantamount to a supplementary school system, and although research by a resident showed there were 3,000 fewer seats in the schools than children in the ward, the local ward boss did not favor a new school. A proposal for a new neighborhood school was blocked in the City Council even though the settlement workers had gotten approval for a new school from the Chicago School Board.

Given these obstacles, Jane Addams encouraged the Hull House Men's Club, a group of residents and young men of the neighborhood interested in politics, to run an independent candidate for alderman, much to the amusement of the local boss. Even though their candidate actually won, the newly elected alderman was unable to resist the opportunities of the situation. It was not too many months before the reform alderman fell into line with the machine.

In the next election, Hull House decided to take on the boss himself. Their candidate was a middle-aged Irish immigrant who was former president of a bricklayer's union. Hull House sponsored a vigorous campaign, focusing on the evils brought to the district by the rule of the "prince of boodlers." While their candidate was easily defeated, he did manage to cut into the usually overwhelming majority the boss ran up. In a third election, in 1898, their candidate was overwhelmingly defeated despite their every effort. Similar campaigns occurred when other settlements fought at the local level, although in some areas settlements did become very powerful factors in local ward politics by holding the balance of power.

Every attempt at intervention is an experiment that reveals the social order, and Hull House discovered a great deal about the realities of life in the ward. By crusading for better streets, or against vice and prostitution in the area, they discovered there was a powerful combine of property owners, bankers, churchmen, and journalists in league with the local political boss.

In one district, defeats at the polls led some of the workers to undertake a study of political sociology at the local level. Here the adolescent street gang was shown to be both a training ground and a source of support for later political leaders. Potential political leaders made their reputations among their peers who later, as adults, joined the local political clubs (Woods, 1898).

Settlement workers also learned that running a workingman in overalls as the people's representative was not the best possible tactic. Many people in the district felt that their representative should stand with the best, and they felt more favorably inclined toward the man who drank champagne and wore a diamond stickpin. When their man received campaign contributions from successful businessmen, it was not a sign of corruption to the voters.

Moreover, they learned that people who supported them during the campaign now expected them to do what the ward leader did: help families get husbands and sons out of jail, provide jobs, and give other favors. They discovered that the private system of political favors served important functions which impartially administered laws could not provide for the people.

Direct political action on the ward level was successful in limited ways and in special circumstances. What was learned about the problems of introducing social change was far more important. Efforts toward political action revealed the organic nature of a community. As the politically active settlement workers came to realize that the neighborhood, the ward, the city, the state, and the nation were inextricably one, the arena of action expanded accordingly.

the settlements, the labor movement, and welfare legislation

The settlement workers not only participated in local municipal reform, but they were an important influence in the often violent labor struggles of that era. Living in working-class neighborhoods, the settlement residents saw that poor working conditions, low pay, and long hours violated human dignity and human welfare. Although they did not intend to involve themselves with the labor movement, it took little time for many settlement workers to become convinced that the human waste and misery they observed were intimately connected with the conditions of industrial capitalism.

The large settlements in Chicago and New York were particularly important in supporting the attempts of workingmen to organize. Initially, the workingmen were not always enthusiastic about receiving help from educated, upper-class youth. Resentment, distrust, and differences in viewpoint concerning what was helpful characterized the relationship between labor leaders and settlement workers. The settlement workers frequently wanted to play the role of mediators in labor disputes, while the laborers wanted allies who were on their side unquestioningly (Addams, 1910; Woods & Kennedy, 1922; Davis, 1959).

The settlement workers made distinct efforts to allay labor's suspicions by helping new locals to organize, by allowing labor unions to meet in the settlements, by organizing discussions, lectures, and conferences; they demonstrated their support of the rights of organized labor in speeches, articles, and books. In some instances they provided active support of strikers by collecting money, by feeding strikers, and by getting economic help for blacklisted labor leaders. Hull House sponsored a cooperative residence for women—the Jane Club—so that women who wished to participate in strikes need not fear they would be put out on the streets (Addams, 1910).

Activity which went beyond simple mediation cost the settlements the financial support of some of their "uptown patrons" who were shocked at what the radicals were doing. Settlement support of labor earned them the enmity of some newspapers who attacked them for harboring anarchists. Some of the settlement leaders were outspoken socialists, but many others favored seeing that the working man got a better share of the wealth, but held no brief for redistributing ownership of the means of production (Woods & Kennedy, 1922; Davis, 1959).

The settlement workers were, in part, responsible for nationwide publicity favorable to the labor cause. In the Chicago stockyard strike of 1904, for example, articles written by settlement workers caused President Theodore Roosevelt to order an investigation of con-

ditions. Further investigations resulted when Upton Sinclair's muckraking novel, *The Jungle*, was published in 1906. Sinclair lived close
by the University of Chicago Settlement while he was gathering
material. He frequently ate at the settlement house and relied on
residents for advice and material for the novel. President Theodore
Roosevelt consulted settlement workers before establishing a commission to investigate conditions. The commission's work resulted in
the federal inspection of meat-packing plants (Davis, 1959).

The settlement workers played a leading role in the fight for laws
regulating child labor and for laws improving working conditions
generally. Not only were they able to arouse public opinion by books,
articles, and speeches to the powerful women's clubs and to church
groups, but they also were active in gathering data concerning industrial abuses. Florence Kelley, an outstanding expert on child labor,
lived at Hull House beginning in 1891, and at Henry Street in 1899.
Her research produced the statistics which influenced legislators to
correct the abuses. While some felt the social workers relied too heavily on numbers—Ben Lindsey called them "scientific robots"—their
numbers produced results because they did not stop with the collection
of data. When Florence Kelley was appointed special investigator for
the Illinois State Bureau of Labor, she had an official base for her
work. Under the provisions of one bill regulating child labor, Florence
Kelley, Alzina Stevens, and Mary Kenney, all settlement workers, were
appointed factory inspectors by reform Governor John Peter Altgeld
(Woods & Kennedy, 1922; Davis, 1959).

This formidable group set out against odds to enforce the bill.
Even though they got few results, and even though the bill was later
declared unconstitutional,[15] they persisted in drafting legislation.
Learning the variety of techniques necessary to achieve meaningful
change, they become experts in the law, and in the use of pressure and
publicity.

Within ten years more effective child labor legislation was passed,

[15] The 1893 bill limited the employment of children under 14 to daylight and to
eight hours. Even though state laws were later passed, the state laws proved weak,
and the settlement workers wanted to obtain stronger federal legislation. In 1904
a National Child Labor Committee was formed, with the settlement movement well
represented. They drew up a model child labor law, and encouraged state campaigns, but they encountered political and philosophical opposition and constitutional obstacles to bills regulating child labor. It was not until much later (really
not until the 1930's) that their efforts were successful (Davis, 1959).

and Jane Addams and her group were instrumental in gaining enforcement of the law through complementary compulsory school attendance laws. The Hull House reformers influenced settlement workers throughout the nation and the fight for laws regulating child labor was carried on in many other states from Massachusetts to California (Woods & Kennedy, 1922).

Lillian Wald suggested the possibility of a Federal Children's Bureau as a coordinating agency to gather data and to make recommendations. The Children's Bureau was born after nine years of labor and a White House Conference on the Care of Dependent Children. It was finally signed into law by President Taft in 1912. Julia Lathrop, a Hull House resident, was appointed its first chief, and Grace Abbott, another Hull House resident, its second.

The settlement workers were instrumental in improving working conditions for women and in promoting the women's trade union movement. The details of the story are not important for our purposes here, but suffice it to say that their efforts were fundamental. As one example, the settlement workers encouraged President Theodore Roosevelt and Congress to pass a bill calling for a federal investigation of the problems of women and children in industry. The Department of Commerce and Labor conducted the investigation, the results of which were published in 19 volumes. These volumes were the major source of information on women and children in industry for many years and were a major resource for reformers in their continuing fight to better the conditions of living and working for all (Davis, 1959).

The role of the settlement workers in developing a variety of social welfare measures is outlined in Woods and Kennedy (1922). Reform of the county poorhouse, relief for the aged, help for the unemployable through sheltered workshops, pensions and day nurseries for widows and their children, studies of living standards, workmen's compensation, and unemployment insurance were all programs which were either initiated by or supported vigorously by settlement workers through the years. These welfare provisions were based upon research and investigations conducted by settlement house residents. The laws were passed in part because of the lobbying of settlement residents. The very content of the laws was suggested by settlement residents who functioned as experts and consultants to legislators and to other governmental officials (Cohen, 1958; Davis, 1959; Pumphrey & Pumphrey, 1961).

the settlements and the Progressive party

For fifty years after the Civil War, but particularly from the 1890's on, there had been a great deal of realignment of social forces, toward the establishment of a more far-reaching democracy. On the political scene there were demands for reform ranging from the fight against corrupt local political bosses to the popular election of senators, a right which was finally achieved in 1913. The campaign for women's rights met increasing success after 1890 (Flexner, 1966). During these years the labor movement was able to call important strikes and to win important concessions from the industrialists. In 1890 the Sherman Anti-Trust Act established means for social control of the activities of the huge corporation. An income tax leveling inequalities of fortune was proposed, supported, and instituted. The definition of what could be supported on a national level under the concept of general welfare was extended greatly.

By 1912, the settlement workers had been in the forefront of the struggle for more than twenty years. Many were convinced that change could be effected only at a national level and in Teddy Roosevelt they felt they had found a candidate who spoke their language. Roosevelt, who had lost the Republican nomination to Taft, became the presidential candidate of the newly formed Progressive party. He drew to him a collection of reformers and idealists, including many of the leaders of the settlement house movement, and many other social workers who by now were cooperating with the settlement workers in efforts to achieve reforms. Despite disquieting questions about others around Roosevelt, the reformers supported him heavily. At the Progressive convention in August of 1912, Jane Addams delivered one of the keynote speeches and seconded Roosevelt's nomination. Raymond Robins, another settlement leader, seconded the nomination of Hiram Johnson as Roosevelt's vice president.

After the convention, many of the settlement workers became heavily involved with the political organization of the Progressive party. They served as political researchers, as ward leaders, as committee chairmen, as speakers, and as candidates for a variety of offices. Jane Addams was a member of the party's national committee, its state committee, and its county committee, and stumped far and wide in support of Progressive candidates.

It was no surprise when Roosevelt lost in 1912; the social workers were disappointed, but ready to continue the party. Many felt the campaign's primary purpose was to educate the public and to prepare the way for a new and more perfect democracy. After the election of 1912, the party continued, and many residents continued the work of political organization in preparation for the next steps. In fact, the Progressive party gained new adherents in the months after the election. Lillian Wald, who had not taken part in the election of 1912, accepted a position on one of the party's committees.

Within months, however, the Progressive party was wracked by factional disputes and personal squabbles. Jane Addams removed herself from the strife and her example was followed by others. Some continued with the Progressive party through the election of 1914, when it lost heavily everywhere. The venture into national politics came to an end. For many, the party's collapse was a sign they could not achieve social reform through direct political action. Later, when the involvement of many of their leaders in the anti-war movement led to their popular vilification, the settlements lapsed into a policy of developing educational, recreational, and group work services in the contemporary professional mold (Davis, 1959).

settlement leaders, the pacifist movement, and World War I

When the war in Europe broke out in 1914, many settlement leaders, particularly Jane Addams, Lillian Wald, and Graham Taylor, became concerned with peace and anti-war movements. While not all settlement workers agreed that international problems were their concern, enough participated to provoke popular reaction against them.

Although Jane Addams was awarded a Nobel Peace Prize in 1931, during the war years and after, she was widely regarded as akin to a traitor and was subject to near violent abuse. The American Legion and the DAR called her un-American. Her protest against conscription and her defense of conscientious objectors, her defense of the "aliens" who were her neighbors in Chicago, and her insistence that war was no way to settle human problems cost her the support of the Women's Clubs. Her actions on behalf of the peace movement and other causes removed from those the developing social work profession had adopted resulted in her isolation, even within the field (Addams, 1910; Linn, 1935). Lillian Wald had similar experiences (Wald, 1915; Duffus, 1935).

After the war, Lillian Wald and Jane Addams were listed as subversives in a report prepared for a senate committee (Duffus, 1935; Linn, 1935). With fears stirred up by the Bolshevik revolution, the settlements, which supported and provided forums for radicals of all kinds, were seen as nests of potentially dangerous subversives. The conservative atmosphere which would not support criticism of the United States during the war years persisted and intensified in the immediate post-war period. Efforts to change social conditions were no longer acceptable (Curti, 1951; Allen, 1959; Davis, 1959).

World War I presented a number of other problems for the settlements. Money was no longer easy to raise. War-related causes, the Red Cross, and similar overseas relief agencies had captured the attention of philanthropists and the settlements received less. Settlement workers spent a great deal of time raising money; eventually many joined the Community Chest and lost their identities as special agencies (Woods & Kennedy, 1922).

Funds for fellowships were cut drastically. No longer could an eager young reformer find support and a place to work through the settlements. Some observers said that the settlement movement had begun to lose its power to attract the young rebels even earlier. Greenwich Village, overseas service, and newer, independent radical movements attracted those who might have gone to live in the settlements. The newer workers coming into the settlements were no longer sparked by deep convictions about social justice. They tended more and more to be professional social workers, trained in case work, social welfare, and community organization. They wanted to help, but they were no longer concerned about social and political action (Davis, 1959).

After the war, some of the leaders turned their attention to international affairs. Jane Addams became very much involved with the Women's International League for Peace and Freedom, and in the next decade spent a great deal of time in overseas travel and at international conferences. Lillian Wald travelled to Europe, Russia, and Mexico during the 1920's. With the older leadership losing its interest, with the changes in the population of the settlement neighborhoods, in the political and social climate, and in the new workers, the settlements, the former "spearheads of reform," became social work agencies in the narrower, contemporary sense of that term. Reform in social work went into its "seedtime." (Chambers, 1965).

summary

The settlement movement began with social need and reached the height of its influence during a period when society was undergoing important changes. It fell back to a less central position when the social order was no longer open to the same kind of changes. As a helping form, the settlement movement was firmly based among those it sought to help, having made its entrance on the basis of immediate, concrete, freely available services which the people who were served both wanted and needed. It maintained its vitality for more than twenty years by drawing upon the energies and ideals of young intellectuals eager to engage themselves with the meaningful problems of the times. The movement had important effects through the local programs implemented, but it had much more far-reaching effects on the larger society both through writings and through efforts to obtain legislative changes at all levels of government. Most importantly, it had a delayed effect as a training ground in reform for those who later took important positions in government. The settlement workers were less successful in their efforts to achieve change through direct political action.

Some may argue with the role the settlements played in achieving change, about whether or not they might have supported more revolutionary social action. Some may argue that the settlement workers were paternalistic, were uplifters, and agents of deviance control who supported a value system and a morality which stifled human development. It can be argued that they were too much involved in Americanization and too much involved in seeing the poor immigrant enter the mainstream of American life to be concerned with the ultimate fate of the mass of people in the hands of big business and big government. It can be argued that they could not really develop local leadership which would have its own class interests at heart, but rather that they served to remove leadership and to direct the interest of the talented toward concern with their own upward mobility. The settlements, it is said, had a one-way view of help, with their own social position and their own moral standards unquestioned and unchanging.

These are important considerations, particularly as the mental health professional and the social scientist (e.g. Gouldner, 1968) turn their attention to the problem of social change in the present day, to the problem of how they can best participate in change. One part of the Black Power movement (Carmichael & Hamilton, 1967) argues that there is no place for the white man, that the white man will protect his own interests, and that his very presence in the struggle emphasizes the black man's inferiority and his inability to help himself.[16] Our recent experience in an agency working with Negro staff strongly suggests that the problem of leadership in helping functions is critical. In those instances in which Negro personnel have not been strong, or have been treated as castrates, they have not taken full leadership positions, and have frequently remained subservient. We have seen many instances, from the earliest days of the poverty program, in which interest in improving one's own social and financial standing grossly interfered with the service function (Sarason et al., 1966). To protect their own positions, workers participated in weak, obviously inadequate programs, or protested them only mildly.

The problem, of course, is not restricted to black personnel, but appears among whites as well, professional and non-professional. The issue is not a simple one of black self-development versus white repression. Rather it seems to us to reflect the more complex issue of the degree to which power can be expected to be used benevolently for the interests of dependent people, when the necessary changes will involve a loss or a sharing of power and position.

The early settlement workers were consciously representative of the best of their own social, cultural, and political traditions. They were uplifters, and they saw their own cultural forms as superior. But it is clear that they respected the traditions of their immigrant neighbors, and urged the immigrant children to know and value the old world culture. It is true they urged upward mobility, but that was, after all, what the immigrants came here to seek. Large numbers of the

[16] Our use of the Black Power issue is meant to be illustrative only. We do not believe that Black Power and white racism are the *only* problems of social change in our contemporary world (see Chapter 11).

immigrants were eager to learn from the settlement workers, did learn from them, and advanced themselves educationally, socially, and economically. There were radicals of all persuasions in the neighborhoods the settlements served and the radical movements gained their own adherents. Choice was available to meet the differing needs of people then, as it should be available now. It is a moral absolutism of its own and a gross oversimplification, which would assert that only a thoroughgoing revolutionary program then would have led to some modern Garden of Eden today, or that such a course was undercut by the commitment of the settlement workers to the American system as they understood it.

Moreover, the viewpoint which asserts that revolutionary change is the only feasible means of achieving true change needs to examine the time perspective of social change. Over time, urban population density, health standards, educational standards, living conditions, and other material benefits have improved. That we continue to have serious concerns about social inequities and about the quality of life means that some old problems continue and new ones are added. It is our feeling that such questions will always be with us, so long as we do not live in a static world.

It is our belief that helping forms are concerned with the quality of life, that the settlement workers understood this very well, and that they acted to improve the quality of life as they understood the concept in terms meaningful to their own day. The settlement movement faltered and lost momentum when it tried to continue its concern with issues which no longer had the significance of earlier years. Perhaps it is asking too much of any social group to recognize that its own central values and its own central goals are not absolute and immutable, and need to change as conditions change.

The lesson that we can take away is that things do change, that it is vital to recognize change, and that it is necessary to accept the diminution if not the demise of the power of older helping forms, as newer forms with newer values evolve to deal with contemporary problems. When helping forms gain power and contribute to cultural lag, become a cultural drag so to speak, then the helping form opens itself to assault. In historical perspective, we cannot see that we can argue with the way in which a helping group defined their problem. We can only learn from it, in order to help to make future forms serve social need more effectively.

6

the visiting teacher—
forerunner of the school social worker

In the past, the child was socialized and educated within the family setting. With social and economic development, the family gave up its function to specialized agencies, one of which was the school. For a time, in colonial America and later, close contact between home and school was maintained. Teachers, largely men, were selected by the community and lived with families. In many small communities teachers commonly rotated among the families of their pupils, receiving their meals as a substantial part of their salaries. During some of the year, teachers worked in the fields side by side with pupils and their families. In the Old South, planters' wives instructed the children of the immediate community (Bailyn, 1960; Atkinson & Maleska, 1964). By 1923, with the exception of kindergartens and specific schools with programs involving home visits, visits by teachers were infrequent (Oppenheimer, 1925).

As the school system became an institution with its own aims and its own culture, the teacher became psychologically isolated from the community,[1] for even under the best of circumstances the interests of teachers and parents are frequently divergent. The teacher is a professional con-

[1] Waller (1932) discusses this point as does Hollingshead (1949). The lives of teachers were frequently regulated in ways the lives of other members of the community were not. Teachers were barred from smoking, drinking, marrying, and other forms of behavior considered natural rights by most adults.

cerned with teaching and with his professional status, while the parent is concerned with the development of his child. As Waller (1932) puts it, ". . . parents and teachers wish the child to prosper in different ways; they wish him well according to different standards of well being" (p. 68). Parents necessarily deal not with neighbors but with agents of the school culture, who necessarily are as concerned with protecting the organization and the prerogatives of the functionaries within the organization as they are with solving the problems of individual children.[2]

The isolation of the school from its surrounding community was exacerbated by the rapid growth of the urban population and the influx of immigrant families with different attitudes toward the school and the schoolteacher. Class sizes of 60 or more and rapid teacher turnover meant that the opportunities for the teacher to know and to understand the child's family and immediate world outside the school building were greatly limited. Furthermore, 68 percent of New York teachers lived more than 50 blocks from their schools (Henderson, 1910–1911). Moreover, the compulsory school laws, and the increased demand that these laws be enforced, brought and kept children in the school system. Where once the school population was essentially self-selected, now it was a mattter of public policy to provide educational services for all children.

We have already discussed the effects such policy had upon the development of special classes, and we have suggested that the reform climate of the period around the turn of the century was instrumental in promoting the development of Witmer's clinic. We shall now describe another clinical service, the visiting teacher, which developed out of the same set of social conditions. a multitude of social problems, a reform climate, and community action. The visiting teacher originated as a means of providing for the child an agent to link school and community.

There is no better way of describing the need for the visiting teacher than to quote from a report by one. Though conditions in the schools prior to 1915 are described, the same statement could apply with little or no modification to today's urban schools.

---

[2] Waller (1932) presents some insightful reports of teachers' and administrators' techniques for dealing with the attempts parents make to influence teachers' treatment of their children in school. He points out that the relationship of parent to teacher is such that a mutually shared problem-solving approach is frequently impossible.

The extension of the influence of the school through the visiting teacher is particularly needed in a city like New York, where the population is heterogeneous and shifting, where the schools are large and congested, and where so many schools are included in one system. The parents of our school children are, many of them, like Angelina's mother, ignorant of the value of education and of the ideals which the school is trying to inculcate. The crowded schools prevent the teachers from giving sufficient individual attention to the children in the classrooms or from influencing to any appreciable degree their homes. The size of the system has made it seem necessary in the past to organize all schools alike, with uniform methods and standards, regardless of the racial and national characteristics which represent widely differing school needs (Johnson, 1916, pp. xiv–xv).

The work of the visiting teacher is not radically new, but rather a very natural extension of the function of the public schools *as a child welfare agency* [italics added] adapted to meet the needs of children in a large municipal organization.

There was a time when the school regarded itself as concerned only with the academic instruction of children under its care, and when social interests and needs were foreign elements not relevant to the big task of education. An inevitable change, however, has come with the changing times.

The doctors and nurses have found their way into the school at the call of the child who is physically unfit for school work; the curriculum has been made to yield to the needs of children who are mentally disqualified; and still there is a group of pupils who seem unable to take their training in wholesale fashion, but need more individualized treatment. They are below standard in scholarship without belonging to the mentally sub-normal class, they are difficult in conduct without being disciplinary cases, and though they avoid truancy they are not in constant attendance.

There are, moreover, the adolescent girls, irritable and neurotic, who are getting poor marks in scholarship and

conduct because they need country care or medical advice,[3]
or perhaps only the understanding sympathy of a friend.
There are the slow girls who have had an increase of home
duties placed on their shoulders at the time when school
demands are also increasing. There are the restless children
who have begun to strain at the tether, whom school does
not interest because it is not as real to them as life outside
its walls and whom the great world of industry will seize
if activities and interests are not provided. There are the
retarded children who are reaching the limit of their mental
development and paying the deferred bills of early mal-
nutrition or heredity, and who are needing special guidance.
Adolescence, individual departure from the accepted average, mental retardation and the urge that sends the boy and
girl out into the world of accomplishment are not phenom-
enal problems. They are ever recurring factors and must
be reckoned with by the schools if opportunity and a chance
for development are to be offered. These, then, are the
children for whom the help of the visiting teacher is enlisted
(Johnson, 1916, pp. 1–2.).

The visiting teacher concept originated out of settlement house work
with children. Sometimes the workers felt the need to be in close
touch with a child's teacher. Located as they were in the community,
the settlement house workers could use their relationship with the
child and his family to assist the school in obtaining the family's
cooperation. The teachers found they obtained a better understanding
of a child when the settlement house worker was able to discuss the
child in another context. As a result of this informal experience, a
resident in each of several settlement houses took on the special
assignment of calling on the families of children who presented special
problems of an educational, social, or medical nature. This worker
came to be known as the school visitor, or visiting teacher.

In all fairness to school administrators, it must be pointed out
that the first visiting teacher was a former schoolteacher, and the

[3] The phrase "country care or medical advice" probably refers to care for patients
with tuberculosis. However, the phrase may be a euphemism for care for unwed
mothers. In Philadelphia the White-Williams Foundation (earlier the Magdalen
Society), organized to help delinquent and wayward girls, was instrumental in the
development of school counselors in the Philadelphia public schools (Oppenheimer, 1925).

work was developed in cooperation with Julia Richman, first woman district superintendant of schools in New York. Moreover, some schoolteachers visited on their own and gave personal charity to a few children. Volunteers from churches and clubs also visited on an informal basis. When the philanthropic societies offered help, principals and teachers were more than happy to refer children to them (Report of the City Superintendant of Schools, New York, 1913–1914). However, the main organizations concerned with formalizing visiting teaching were the settlement houses and the Public Education Association of New York.

One of the guiding spirits of visiting teaching was Miss Mary Marot, a former teacher who believed the schools were a prime medium for far-reaching social reform. In the fall of 1906, the settlement houses formed a committee to supervise the work of two visitors in three school districts. A few months later, the Public Education Association of New York became interested in the movement and absorbed the Visiting Teacher Committee started by the settlement house workers. By the fall of 1907, the Public Education Association hired Miss Jane Day as a visiting teacher on a full-time basis.[4] She worked closely with Julia Richman. By the academic year 1911–1912, seven workers were employed. The Public Education Association publicized the visiting teacher work in order to persuade the Board of Education to adopt the service in the schools. In 1913, the New York Board of Education allocated funds to establish a visiting teacher service within the city system.

The visiting teacher service began in somewhat similar fashion about 1906 in several other cities. In Boston, the Women's Education Association first employed a home and school visitor for one school. Other private groups such as neighborhood associations and the Boston Home and School Association placed visitors in additional districts over the next few years. Settlement houses picked up the work by providing staff members to carry out home and school visiting in their immediate districts. In Hartford visiting teachers assisted the school psychologist in obtaining histories and they carried out the recommendations of

---

[4] The role of women in a variety of reforms was obviously very important. We have already pointed out the role of women in introducing social reforms and in establishing the juvenile court. Here is another instance in which an important innovation, deriving from a reform philosophy, originated with educated women in this pre-World War I period. Almost all of the early visiting teachers were women. The stamp they put on the field is still fresh today.

the psychological clinic at home and in school.[5] In Philadelphia, various private associations provided workers to do home investigating, sometimes as part of the attendance service, in an effort to enforce the compulsory education laws. In other communities, women's clubs and even private citizens were instrumental in beginning visiting teacher work and in influencing boards to adopt the service permanently. Vocational and educational guidance services were established as part of the same movement in Philadelphia and Chicago. From 1913 on, many public school systems appointed their own visiting teachers.

An impetus to the spread of the visiting teacher was provided by the Commonwealth Fund's Program for the Prevention of Delinquency, adopted in 1921, which we shall discuss in greater detail in connection with the establishment of child guidance clinics. This program was organized on the premise that early contact with children within the schools could be used to prevent delinquency and maladjustment. The Commonwealth Fund, working through the Public Education Association, established a National Committee on Visiting Teachers which placed thirty visiting teachers in thirty communities for a three-year demonstration. Additional funds were provided for visiting teachers by the Bureau of Children's Guidance, a psychiatric clinic within the school system connected with the New York School of Social Work. The Bureau of Children's Guidance and the New York School undertook the professional training of visiting teachers during the bureau's existence.

The Public Education Association continued to maintain a demonstration staff which conducted research on children's problems in the schools and on the work of the visiting teacher. Concern for evaluation of the work was present from the beginning; Johnson's report (1916) contains a detailed study of the first few years' operation. Evaluation research was part of the effort to stimulate school interest in adoption of the service. As we have pointed out, the early social workers had an important commitment to research as a tool for stimulating social change. Job descriptions for the visiting teacher frequently included research to determine the needs of children in the schools (Oppenheimer, 1925).

Within a relatively few years after the beginning of the service, public school systems took over the demonstration programs. From

[5] Witmer had long used social workers in a similar capacity in his clinic.

that point onward, the history of the visiting teacher movement illustrates the problem in innovating services within the school system.

This discussion will become clearer to the reader if we consider the actual clinical work of the visiting teacher. Clinical work brought the visiting teacher into direct contact, and sometimes direct conflict, with the organizational structure of the school system. The visiting teachers had a theory of behavior disorder and of therapy which was largely situational in nature.

> The function of the visiting teacher is the adjustment of conditions in the lives of individual children, to the end that they may make more normal or more profitable school progress. These adjustments may be made in the school, in the home, or in the environment, wherever there proves to be an adverse condition responsible for school conduct, scholarship or attendance, or influencing it to a greater or less extent (Johnson, 1916, p. 3).

When she began her work with a school, the visiting teacher would familiarize herself with the ethnic character of the neighborhood, the standard of living, the attitudes of the people toward education, housing conditions, the predominant industries in which parents worked, recreational opportunities, special educational programs in school and out, and the availability of the services of public and private agencies. These were the resources and liabilities of the neighborhood, resources the visiting teacher would employ in making adjustments in the child's interest, and liabilities she would interpret to the school in order to elicit a more sympathetic view of the child's problem.[6]

It is apparent from various statements that the effectiveness of the visiting teacher was a function of her understanding of a particular school situation. There are also several allusions to problems visitors encountered in the schools. Some may have stemmed from the goals some of the visiting teachers held for their own work. They felt, even

[6] We shall return to the task of interpreting the child's situation to the school, for it seems to be a function rediscovered by every group which attempts to develop a consulting relationship with the school and the classroom teacher. Wickman (personal communication) mentions it as a primary value in the relationship of the early child guidance clinics to the schools and Sarason, et al. (1966) devote considerable attention to the same issue in Chapter 7, "Helping The Teacher Change Her Perception of a Problem."

at that early date, that the needs of individuals were frequently subordinated to the needs of the school (Johnson, 1916). The early visiting teachers made suggestions concerning curriculum, school organization, and methods of teaching, and some complained that the system was too unyielding to individual needs (National Association of Visiting Teachers, 1921). The specific problems were not spelled out in any sources we have seen, but they seem to have been attitudes with which help was given and received, attitudes toward the delegation of authority, and attitudes toward modifying the school situation.

Oppenheimer (1925) states that principals in difficult areas were chosen for their social mindedness, and that such social-minded principals were quick to recognize the value of visiting teacher work. By implication, some were not social minded and did not quickly grasp the significance of the work. There were suggestions that visiting teachers should not be placed in schools where the principals were unreceptive. Despite conflicts, word of the value of the service spread through the New York system until, within ten years after its beginning, there were requests from over 175 school principals (Johnson, 1916).

The visiting teachers had "port-of-entry" difficulties (Sarason, et al., 1966), but the pressure of school problems facilitated the development of the service. It was no accident that the visiting teacher service was initiated in what we would today call a "lower-class" or inner-city school. Sarason, et al. (1966) also found that a clinical service was more readily received in an embattled urban system than in a suburban system. The suburban system had children with problems, but did not have the same pressures upon it. When we see that clinical services typically have had the same difficulties in establishing working relationships with the public schools (Allen, 1929; Ridenour, 1948; Grant & Stringer, 1964; Sarason, et al., 1966), we feel it is a real loss that the early clinical researchers did not identify and describe the problems in relating to the school system.

Once the visiting teacher entered the school, she had to develop working relationships with the faculty. It soon became apparent it was better for all concerned if the visiting teacher concentrated her efforts in one school and was viewed as a member of the staff. However, her ability to influence the situation depended on herself: " . . . she could never work out her plans for the children under her care by the force of any authority she might be given over them or over the teachers. She can be effective in a school only as she can make the teachers realize that she understands their problems, and that if her work is primarily to help the children and give them a fuller opportunity, that help must be given in such a way that it will be felt to be an assistance, not a hindrance in the classroom and in the principal's office" (Johnson, 1916, p. 8). This admonition, statements that above all a visiting teacher needed tact, the veiled and not-so-veiled criticisms of aspects of the school program, and instances in which the visitor's recommendations differed from the teacher's imply that there was some difficulty in relationships with teachers. By and large the visiting teachers were able to establish good working relationships within the schools, but they are not explicit enough about their problems to afford us helpful examples.

One wonders whether the fact that the reports were authored under the auspices of the agencies which supported the original services had anything to do with the glossing over of difficulties. If there were more problems than were presented, the contemporary community mental health movement is the poorer by the loss of the information.

How did the visiting teacher operate? In two ways: first, working to develop programs to deal with general problems of the school and the community; and second, dealing with the needs of individual children. The first method of operation appears to have developed only in the early years, and by the 1921 report (National Association of Visiting Teachers, 1921) little further mention is made of organizational work in the community. By 1921, concepts of case work were becoming current, and the visiting teachers, identifying themselves as social workers, began to seek training in casework, psychoanalysis, psychiatry, mental hygiene, and even mental testing. What was thought of as social service by the settlement house workers seems to have disappeared in favor of casework with individuals. We shall return to treatment by environmental manipulation and quote from case studies of that day, but let us first describe some of the programmatic work and some of the concepts the early visiting teachers held.

The visiting teachers engaged in diverse activities, for the work was an experiment and could develop flexibly. They worked out a variety of clubs and classes to meet the needs both of children with whom they had been working and of other children. Classes included special assistance in schoolwork, dramatics, athletics, handicrafts, and reading clubs, dancing classes, and excursions. Clubs to foster social relationships between younger and older children were developed. Housekeeping classes were established for some younger girls. The visiting teachers also helped arrange for systematic programs of clinical examination, medical treatment within the school, and even special diets for poorly nourished children. In some schools, programs for psychometric evaluation of retarded children were initiated through the efforts of the visiting teacher. Educational efforts in the community were carried out through lectures at parents' meetings and appearances at teacher conferences. Some worked to form school and neighborhood associations. The extension of a variety of special classes, the wider use of the school building, and the school lunch service were wholly or in part the consequence of the visiting teachers' activity.

The early visiting teachers, reflecting as they did the orientation of the settlement house, envisioned within each school a social service department to supervise the visiting teachers and be responsible in an organizational sense to the principal of the school. All community-oriented activities, including the formation of student groups, parent groups, neighborhood associations, and all relationships with outside social agencies and community organizations would be the responsibility of this department. Experimentation with the school as a social center, the development of after-school clubs and classes, and even vocational programs would fall within the aegis of the service. Research, including social surveys of the neighborhood and the school, would be another function. In an important sense the Gary School (Chapter 7) was the fulfillment of this dream, but in later writings about the visiting teacher little further mention is made of the broad social service department. The reader may be interested in comparing New Haven's Community School concept (Community Progress, Inc., 1966), a contemporary development to meet the human problems of urban poverty, with the Gary School concept, and with the vision of the early visiting teachers.

As we have indicated, in work with the individual child, the visiting teacher used a situational theory. She would obtain a referral from the teacher through the principal, discuss the problem with the teacher, observe in class, interview the child in school, and then visit at home.[7]

---

[7] Those of us (Sarason, et al., 1966) who have worked in inner-city schools have been astonished at the remarkable similarity in the approach we evolved to that used by the visiting teachers. The problems and the solutions are similar enough to reinforce our belief that common circumstances lead to common concepts.

The visiting teachers, at least in their early days, observed no working hours, but would call on families at night or on Saturdays, if need be, to see working parents.

The visitor tried to determine "which of the conditions found have been most instrumental in causing the difficulty, or in hindering the necessary adjustment." The fundamental difficulties were divided roughly into seven areas:

> 1. *school maladjustment* ("When school conditions seem to be definitely responsible for his failure to come up to a standard or when a modification of requirements adjusts his difficulty");
> 2. *lack of family cooperation* (neglect, suspicion of school, poor parental educational standards);
> 3. *economic stress;*
> 4. *ill health;*
> 5. *immoral family conditions* (drunkenness, physical violence, sexual irregularities);
> 6. *adverse neighborhood conditions* (gangs, disorderly houses, cheap shows);
> 7. *individual peculiarity* (social maladjustment, mental unsuitability for school life, exceptional instability).

The cases of "individual peculiarity" constituted about 4 percent of referrals in the school year 1913–1914 (Johnson, 1916).

The visiting teacher interpreted the child's behavior to the school in order to achieve modifications in the school's behavior toward the child.

> *Example 1:* A teacher found an eighth-grade child cheating at her lessons. The visiting teacher investigated the situation and discovered the child was waiting tables and washing dishes in the evenings to earn money for a graduation dress. She told the teacher, who realized the child's behavior was a means of doing her schoolwork, not avoiding it. The visitor then made arrangements to obtain money for the child, and helped her to get a tutor and a scholarship, which enabled her to go on to high school.
> *Example 2:* Angelina, a third-grade child, was referred for constant lateness and indifference in school. The visitor

discovered the child was working at home sewing, not because the family was in need, but because the mother believed this was proper for an Italian girl. The visitor
helped to persuade the mother that her child's education
was important, and she encouraged the teacher to be lenient
about the lateness while mother was being educated to
education. Instead of being punished for lateness, Angelina
was commended for improvement by the teacher. She
started her days in school in a better frame of mind. With
continued attention and stimulation from the teacher and
the visitor, the child's work improved until she was placed
in a rapid advancement class where she did two years' work
in one.

In these examples and in others, the visiting teacher was able to
glean information which put the child's behavior in a new light for
the classroom teacher. While it is apparent that the visiting teacher
had the time to seek explanations for the child's behavior and that the
classroom teacher did not, it is also apparent that the classroom teachers
tended not to think in terms of causes of behavior.

The visiting teachers sometimes recommended a change of class
as a way of handling a problem.

Example 3: Anna had fits of temper in her fifth-grade
classroom, refusing to work and throwing her books on the
floor. The visiting teacher enlisted the child's interest and
that of her teacher in keeping a "self-control" book, which
the child brought to the visiting teacher each time they met.
The procedure worked well for two months, when again
friction arose in the classroom. The child was transferred to
another class where she worked well and gave no trouble.

There are several cases reported of precocious children whose
problem was solved by promotion.

Example 4: For three years, Sam gave all his teachers
except the dramatic teacher the impression he was dull. He
was a disciplinary case frequently reported to the principal.

His teachers thought him feebleminded, but when the visiting teacher's investigation showed that out of school he made friends with engineers and mechanics who taught him about machines and allowed him to run engines and motors, she gave him an intelligence test.[8] He rated so high that she suggested he be advanced two grades. This was done and he immediately began to improve. There were no more shamings in school or trips to the principal's office except to show a good report card. Sam had found his proper level (Johnson, 1919, p. 32).

Special class situations were sometimes used as a temporary means of helping a child with a problem. When no special class existed, visiting teachers often encouraged the development of such classes to provide for children with a variety of problems, not just the retarded.

The transfer of children from one classroom to another (discussed in some detail by Sarason, et al., 1966) and from one teacher to another is often the fastest and most effective form of help. This was a discovery the visiting teachers had made, and it is a discovery which has been lost to a generation of mental health workers who have been taught concepts of intrapsychic supremacy exclusively.

What is missing from the case vignettes, for there are few full case studies available, is a detailed description of how the visiting teachers became influential enough to recommend changes of class, and what interpersonal and organizational problems they encountered. It is possible that the visiting teachers had approaches which permitted such transfers without any strain. It is also possible that with classes of 50 and 60, one child more or less is not missed by a teacher.

The method most frequently employed by the visiting teachers was called "supervision." Supervision involved more than seeing the child for a few interviews. The visitor took a personal interest in the child, meeting him at school and at home, sharing his interests, and helping him to realize the visitor wished to share his successes

---

[8] There are several references to these early visiting teachers administering intelligence tests, but no such references later on. Some of the special class programs and some of the psychological services associated with school systems had their own visiting teachers, but there is no indication they administered tests. It is not clear whether they received training in psychometrics, or whether some were psychologists.

and prevent his failures. The relationship frequently continued for a period of years.

The help that was provided was concrete, personal, and exhaustive.

> *Example 5:* Nine-year-old Sadie had a bad reputation, was neglected, disheveled, and often fell asleep in school. Home visits soon established that her mother lived away from her home at her place of employment. Her father drank heavily, and he and the child slept together in the only bed. The visitor helped Sadie's mother make arrangements to be home more often, and arranged for the child to have lunch money. The visitor taught the child to fix her hair, gave her hair ribbons and dresses, and made it a point to inspect her frequently. She arranged for a tutor at the nearby settlement and helped to program the hours after school. The neighborhood librarian took an interest in Sadie, she joined a club at the settlement house, and was admitted to a gym class after the visitor obtained the proper shoes and costume. A kindly neighbor took the child in when the parents were away. All of this attention resulted in a marked transformation. Sadie's appearance changed and she began to bring perfect papers for the visiting teacher to see. Apparently the family situation also cleared up considerably, but it is not clear why.

The visitors intervened with the courts, social agencies, and welfare services on behalf of the child. They helped in obtaining employment, grants for special purposes, clothes, and scholarships, including funds which would enable a child to feel he was contributing to his family while he stayed in high school. They helped arrange for participation in organizations such as the Boy Scouts. The visitors frequently acted as school counselors, helping the students to select their courses. Sometimes the relationship to the visitor prevented the student from leaving school. The visiting teachers apparently used tutors, including high school students, to help younger children individually or in groups. Sometimes the tutor was instructed to minimize the formal academic content of the sessions. Volunteers from Big Brothers and Big Sisters were used extensively as companions for children.

Psychotherapeutic methods were not yet developed, but some of the cases indicate that the visiting teachers permitted some ventilation of personal conflicts, such as guilt over masturbation. Where the visiting teacher felt the problem called for a specialist's help, she made a referral to the appropriate source. As we shall see when we discuss the early child guidance clinics, the visiting teachers cooperated very closely with the specialist, providing observations about the child at home, in school, and in his neighborhood, and carrying out the specialist's directions. At this early date, the visiting teachers did not complain about a lack of communication with the specialists.

It is also important to note the variety of symptoms and complaints treated by the situational approach outlined above. Not only were neglected and dependent children treated in this manner; children exhibiting behavioral disorders also seemed to be helped. Temper tantrums, incorrigibility, shyness and inarticulateness, apparent feeblemindedness, underachievement, indifference, impertinence, neglect of personal appearance, parental overprotection, truancy, lying, stealing, fearfulness, excessive daydreaming, and adolescent oversensitivity were also treated successfully.

Such outcome studies as there are in the early literature indicate that some 92 percent of the cases were improved or partially improved, according to the judgment of the visiting teacher. There was a significant improvement in grades among children helped by the visiting teacher (compared to those from the same classrooms matched to the treated cases and neither referred nor treated). Since the treated cases were referred as problems and controls were not, the finding is quite remarkable (Oppenheimer, 1925). This early experience provides a challenge for those in the mental health professions who regard office psychotherapy as the treatment preferred for the variety of symptoms we mentioned.

We will conclude this section with a typical case vignette which illustrates the methods of treatment carried out over a period of years.

> The case of Miriam is one in point. She was in a 6B grade. The principal reported her as incorrigible, with a tendency toward immorality, unruly in the classroom, untruthful, and untidy in appearance, and asked the visitor to take her out of school and send her to work. When the visiting teacher called at the home she found that Miriam's mother had died a short time before, leaving Miriam in

charge of the household which consisted of her father who was out of work and two brothers. She cooked the meals, washed the clothes, and took the place of the mother.

Of a highly sensitive nature, very retiring and backward, she made few girl friends. She was untruthful, but she told tales to win sympathy. She was on the street at night, and while she did not seek companions of the lower type, they came to her, using her as a shield to cover some of their wrongdoings.

The visiting teacher became very friendly with Miriam and found new friends for her, and the old ones were given up. Through the assistance of a relief organization, the family was moved to better quarters. Work was secured for the father, and the younger brother was placed in a Hebrew class in a neighborhood organization.

When Miriam was promoted to the seventh grade the visiting teacher watched her closely. She asked that the child should be given to an especially sympathetic teacher to whom she told the story of her home life.

Throughout two years, the visiting teacher followed her progress. The child came to her with all sorts of problems, now a discouraging mark in school work, now household cares that needed school help for their adjustment and again financial difficulties caused by the unemployment of her father or brother. Tutoring was provided, arrangements were made to excuse her a little early so that she could prepare the evening meal for the Jewish Sabbath; and plans for tiding the family over a period of stress were worked out with the agency for relief.

Gradually, Miriam showed the result of this friendly supervision. The dime novels which had been her choice and rough friends ceased to satisfy her, and when she graduated she had won the affection of the finest girls in her class, and the genuine respect of her teachers. All trace of immoral tendency disappeared (Johnson, 1916, p. xi).

The remainder of the history of the visiting teacher movement is the story of changes after its introduction into the public school system. Clinical services are shaped as much by their settings as they are by the guiding concepts the professionals employ in their work. Moreover, the period of greatest growth of the visiting teacher movement was in the 1920's, a period in which the predominant social forces and the mood of the country were vastly different from those of the twenty years preceding the First World War. The fact that the visiting teacher movement was encapsulated by the system it meant to change should be considered by those in community mental health who hope to influence other system and agencies to change.

From the very beginning, the sponsoring agency saw itself conducting a demonstration of a service which would be adopted by the public school system once it had demonstrated its worth. Innovations sponsored by private philanthropy are frequently structured as temporary affairs which will be financed on a permanent basis by local or public agencies. In this shift from private, outside support to public inside support lies an important force which helps to change the service. In this case, as public support increased, a good deal of the literature and the interest shifted from a consideration of the work itself to a consideration of the place of the work within the school system. Johnson's (1916) report contains little discussion of administrative problems. The later reports of the National Association of Visiting Teachers (1921) and of Oppenheimer (1925) devote a great deal of attention to administrative, organizational, and professional issues, and relatively little attention to the theory and the details of professional practice.

In the case of the visiting teacher, the settlement houses and the Public Education Association supported the service for about seven years after it was begun. Although the superintendent of schools in New York was in favor of the work, he had to include requests for funds in his budget for several years before the Board of Education was willing to hire its own visiting teachers. The first seven visiting teachers, supported by the Board of Education, were placed under the direction of an associate superintendent of schools. Almost immediately discussion of supervision, cooperation with other departments, hours, case loads, record keeping, and qualifications of education and experience, appeared.

The organization of the National Association of Visiting Teachers, beginning in 1916, contributed discussions of standards of training and practice. (Eventually the group was absorbed into the National Association of Social Workers as the School Social Workers Section.)

By 1921, the visiting teachers themselves felt they had developed "a real technique of social case work as applied to the schools and that this technique is only acquired by training plus experience." The training plus experience considered desirable by the National Association leaders included graduation from a four-year college with a background in education, one year's training in social work, and two years' grade school teaching experience. Salaries in most systems were based upon the scale for grade school teachers, and so a person with such training might find herself earning less than high school teachers in the same system.

The National Committee on Visiting Teachers, which attempted to conduct demonstration programs in thirty cities, apparently had difficulty recruiting people with the requisite background. They recognized that from a practical viewpoint it would be almost impossible to obtain people with the desirable qualifications, and so proposed that minimum qualifications should include graduation from a two-year teacher training course, one year's teaching experience, and one year's work in an approved school of social work. Many systems, in their desire to have a home and school visitor, selected classroom teachers from within the system, or employed people who had the qualifications to be appointed as teachers.

The practicalities of the situation resulted in a shift toward people who would follow an accepted course of training and away from the "mavericks" who were attracted into the work in the earliest days. In discussing the settlement house movement we noted the motivations which seemed to be characteristic of those who entered the settlement houses. A sizeable percentage of the very earliest of the visiting teachers must have been people similar to the settlement workers. One survey of their educational backgrounds, when there were no more than a hundred people in the field, showed that of those with college degrees, many had received them at "name" schools. Barnard, Bryn Mawr, Simmons, Smith, Vassar, Wells, Teachers College, Columbia, Clark, the University of Chicago, New York University were their colleges; just a sprinkling of the state universities were represented (National Association of Visiting Teachers, 1921).

It seems inconceivable that women entering the field after attending normal schools in pursuit of conventional careers as teachers would be of the same intellectual calibre, or have the same social outlook, as the educated upper-class women of the early 1900's who were the backbone of the feminist and other reform movements of the day.

By the 1920's efforts toward social reform had all but died. In the social work field, professional training became heavily influenced by psychiatric and psychoanalytic thinking because of the development of schools of psychiatric social work. Case work was formalized and the "social service" of an earlier day became less important to the professionally trained worker. No longer was the visiting teacher an agent of reform of society or of reform within the school system itself. With changes in the times and changes in professional practice, social workers had narrowed to a focus on the inner psychological problems of individuals.

7

the Gary schools—
the prevention of alienation

The problem of alienation was foremost among the concerns of many social reformers and intellectuals at the turn of the century. A variety of efforts were made to combat the social problems of the day by changing or creating institutions, many of which, at least in their early days, were closely intertwined with community life. The visiting teacher represented one effort to change an institution by linking home, school, and community. The progressive education movement, a product of the 19th and early 20th centuries, was designed to make education more relevant to an industrial society. It is not our purpose to recount the history of the movement or the reasons for its success. That has been done very well by Cremin (1964). However, in the sense that the progressive education movement was designed to help the individual be more competent in his social environment and achieve personal fulfillment, the movement can be said to represent a mental health effort in the community.

Progressive education and the reform movement in the schools produced no more complete model than the public schools of Gary, Indiana. Developed in 1906, under the leadership of the superintendent of schools, William Wirt, the Gary schools reflected John Dewey's influence. The school was to be both an intimate society and an extended community. Within the school, teachers and pupils would be closely related; the school would also function as a social and cultural center for the surrounding population.

Though it may be going a little far afield to discuss the Gary schools in detail, since they cannot claim even distant ancestry to later clinical services, to the degree that the community mental health movement involves itself with institutional reform, the Gary schools have relevance to us today. In the Gary story we find a cure for the malaise that grips urban schools and we find ideas far in advance of those underlying developments such as the community school and the skill center program built in New Haven in the 1960's (Community Progress, Inc., 1966).

William Wirt sold the idea of the Gary School as a practical expedient for solving some of the educational problems of Gary, Indiana. At the time Gary was a steel town, growing rapidly from the barren sand dunes and struggling to assimilate the immigrant laborers required by industrial growth. Because Wirt had the advantage of developing a new system rather than rebuilding an old one, he was able to propose curricular and organizational innovation. The school board found appealing his plans for a better education and a more efficient use of the educational dollar.

Wirt built schools which contained, in addition to regular classrooms, a number of specialized facilities, including an auditorium, gyms, swimming pools, shops, laboratories, art studios, and luncheon facilities. There was a great deal of surrounding acreage suitable for gardening and farming, parks and playgrounds. Wirt pointed out that by doing away with the concept of a classroom for each teacher and a seat for each child, by using a platoon system, and by using all of the classrooms and specialized facilities all of the time, a school could accommodate twice as many children on a full-time basis. To reduce discontinuity in education, the school building contained cultural facilities such as libraries and museums. The school was open to adults in the community for recreation and education and was intimately tied to other community agencies such as the YMCA and the churches. Wirt developed the released-time concept for religious education as part of his program of involving the school with the community. The school day, the school week, and the school year were all extended; the school became a year-round community facility.

Within the school, all work, study, and play converged to create not a preparation for life, but a life in itself, much as the old household was a life in itself. The concept was implemented not only by providing all facilities within the school, but by making the actual academic work of the school real and vital. In the Gary school, repair, decoration, and improvement of the school were part of the educational program. Skilled workers were the shop teachers. They were chosen for their abilities in carpentry, plumbing, cabinetry, sheet metal work, printing, and electricity, and for their personal traits. All maintenance, repair, and building were carried out by these men; they did the work of the school community assisted by older students who functioned almost as apprentices. Each of the shops was used as a teaching facility for younger children who came to help the older ones and to be taught by them. This system extended to academic classes as well. Distance between faculty and students was reduced by use of student assistants.

Shop projects were the school's real work and its method of education. In the lunchroom the children learned to cook by preparing meals which were sold on a profit-sharing basis to faculty and children. The children learned arithmetic, accounting, and business and secretarial skills by keeping records of the school's business activities. In some instances, grades were replaced by token wages which the children earned. In sewing classes children made clothes for themselves and their families. They learned to make and repair shoes because it was discovered that many poor parents could not provide them. In botany and zoology classes, they took charge of the gardens, the lawns, and the school zoo. It is important to emphasize that children of all ages participated in the work, and that all the shops and laboratories had generous expanses of window so that everyone who was curious could see what was happening inside. Nothing was hidden; every activity was open to all in some form.

A central aspect of the Gary school was the auditorium, which in one instance contained a stage large enough to hold an athletic contest. Each child spent one hour a day in the auditorium, younger and older children at the same time. The teachers were responsible for arranging each day's program in cooperation with their pupils. Some part of the auditorium program was devoted to a presentation of an aspect of school life. Specialty teachers discussed their work, children debated about school life, exhibited schoolwork, or put on plays they sometimes wrote themselves. The auditorium was meant to be a community theatre in which the children shared all the school's activities.

Within the general structure of the school system, a strong attempt was made to individualize the program. Dewey and Dewey (1915) described how children could emphasize their strengths, compensate for weaknesses, and proceed at an individual pace. The attempt to tailor make programs was in part designed to provide for "even the most difficult pupil," so that instead of dropping out or failing, each could find something for himself in the school.

Discipline was to come primarily from the sense of involvement with the school itself and only secondarily from the teacher's authority. Interest in the work was to help sustain order, while the emphasis on the teacher as a helper was to eliminate the teacher's role as an arbitrary disciplinarian. Some observers felt the children wanted to come to school so badly that the threat of being sent home was sufficient to enforce order. The school attempted to create an atmosphere where children could enjoy learning, but children did not come to school solely to play, as some critics charged. Many came to school voluntarily on Saturdays, Sundays, and during the summers to do their schoolwork under the guidance of their regular teachers.

For a few, the more vigorous attention of the school principal was necessary, and others who could not adapt to the school were sent to the school farm, which had a model dairy, good orchards, and numerous farm buildings on a hundred acres. The farm was run by a young agriculturist who employed scientific methods. The boys who went there built their own living quarters and clubroom, worked and were paid for their work, and paid for room and board out of their earnings. A teacher was provided who integrated formal schooling with the farm work. Eventually the boys either returned to the school or obtained employment.

There were no extra-curricular activities in the schools. Fraternities did not develop. All of the school teams, clubs, the school paper, the orchestra and glee clubs were integral parts of the formal educational program. Students engaged in active political campaigns and elections; there were student councils and civic improvement societies.

Because the schools were completely equipped, they served as community educational and recreational facilities on evenings and weekends. The Gary evening schools had an attendance which was two-thirds that of the day schools, a figure confirmed by the school's critics. All courses authorized by state law were offered and all shops and laboratories, studios, and classrooms were thrown open to the public. Special courses were designed to correlate evening school work with the needs of local industry.

Both adults and children were given full and free use of the recreational facilities. The gyms, pools, and playgrounds were almost always open and playgrounds were lit so that they could be used at night. Social, political, and neighborhood organizations used the school's facilities, presenting films and lectures and holding innumerable community forums, group meetings, and conferences. Parents brought their children with them when they attended evening classes or meetings in the school and the children were allowed to play freely. In the truest sense, the public schools became "schools for the public."

Teachers were relatively self-directed because they were less compelled to follow rigid curricula. The overall head of the school system was the superintendent. An executive principal was in charge of each school. He was responsible for scheduling, for supervising pupils' schedules, maintaining discipline, and for other ordinary administrative work. He was not responsible for the educational program.

Supervisors of instruction in cooperation with the teachers developed curricula and promoted or demoted children. All the industrial and manual training shops were under a director of industrial work who also supervised repair and maintenance. The teacher-workmen in the shops were responsible to him. Each building also had a head manual training teacher who not only supervised the industrial classes but also acted as a vocational advisor for the children. Teachers in the various academic divisions were designated assistant supervisors of instruction and were responsible for coordinating courses in their subjects. Teachers under them were specialists in subject matter and many taught both elementary and high school level classes. Each taught a subject to a different group each hour.

In addition to the subject matter specialists, there were application teachers who met their classes in the shops and studios. They were expected to consult with the subject matter specialists so that they could teach subject matter through application. An application teacher was the head of a group of eight teachers and was responsible for correlating the work of various classes.

Teachers were also classed as head teachers and assistants according to their level of experience. The head teacher in each classroom supervised the assistant teacher. New teachers were initiated in this fashion, so that a constant spirit of in-service training was maintained.

Instead of employing visiting teachers, the Gary system gave responsibility for the work to a register teacher. The register teacher was the faculty advisor, the disciplinary and sociological overseer for a geographic area with some fifty families. All the children in the area met with the register teacher for a weekly general conference. Monthly reports, problems in discipline, attendance, and other issues were channeled through the register teacher, who was expected to meet with the parents in school or to make home visits as necessary.

The burden on the teacher was large, but it was relieved in a number of ways. First, the teachers were given time to do their preparation and other administrative work during the school day. The pupil assistants helped with many classroom chores such as grading papers.

Second, the teachers were paid additional money for any time they taught in the evening, weekend, or summer school. Their earnings were substantially above those of New Yory City teachers.

Third, the importance of teachers was emphasized when they were asked to train people from other schools who wished to learn the Gary system. A visitor was assigned to a teacher as an assistant and learned by doing in the classroom. The visitor paid a fee which went to the instructing teacher.

Fourth, the teachers were given a great deal of leeway in the conduct of their classes. Educational innovation was encouraged and rigid adherence to curricula or materials was not demanded. Supervisory control was minimized; the teacher was permitted to work out his own creative methods. Considerable overlap in function was allowed and auditorium programs informed the teachers of what was happening in the school. Communication, involvement, and maximum self-direction were encouraged by the system.

The Gary system received a great deal of popular and professional attention. It was in keeping with the spirit of the times. Educators from all over the country visited Gary. Our description of the Gary schools is taken largely from Bourne's (1916) book; Bourne also published a series of articles about the Gary schools in the *New Republic.* John Dewey, who wrote about the Gary school in *Schools of Tomorrow* (Dewey & Dewey, 1915), gave the system his personal blessing. Numerous school systems throughout the country adopted some features of the Gary school program. Wirt himself wrote and spoke extensively (Wirt, 1912), was consultant to the New York City schools, and devised a program which was actually implemented in a number of schools in the Bronx. A preliminary report of the experience in one New York school is provided by Taylor (1916).[1]

While the Gary experiment was greeted enthusiastically by many, some of whom observed it only superficially, the experiment also had its critics. Some criticism came from professional educators who were appalled at what they saw as a lack of discipline in the classrooms. They objected that often the shop teachers had no formal training. Some critics, interested only in the economics of the system, did not address themselves to the spirit of the venture. In making recommendations to their own board, the committee from Syracuse (1915), for example, suggested that various parts of the Gary system such as platooning could be adopted in Syracuse, but they did not approve the whole system.

A more thorough examination of the Gary schools is found in the report by Flexner and Bachman (1918). The General Education Board of New York City, a Rockefeller-funded agency interested in the study of education, was commissioned by the Gary Board of Education and by Superintendent Wirt to do a thorough evaluation of the Gary schools. The report was published in eight volumes. The Flexner and Bachman (1918) volume contains an overview of the survey and a summary of the General Education Board's findings and recommendations.

While the report praised the concepts involved in the schools, it was extremely critical of many phases of the plan's execution. In particular, Flexner and Bachman felt that the loose supervisory and administrative structures made for confusion rather than progress. They felt that the execution of such a bold plan required the most exacting attention to detail, attention which was not present in the

---

[1] The attempt to introduce the Gary system into New York City provides one of the very important case histories of the problems of large-scale social and institutional change. The "Garyizing" of the New York schools became an issue in the mayoralty election of 1917. In October, 1917, just before the election, there was a week-long riot in the Bronx, Brooklyn, and upper Manhattan. The children broke windows, fought the police, and supported by their parents, tried to spread the strike to uninvolved schools. At the height of the disturbance, ten thousand people demonstrated on the streets. John Purroy Mitchel, the incumbent fusion mayor, was badly defeated, partly because he advocated the Gary plan. The detailed story will be presented in a volume devoted to the Garyizing of the New York schools which we are currently writing.

Gary schools. As a result, the required integration of practical and academic work was not really achieved; too many of the teachers, left on their own, simply reverted to teaching by the methods they had been taught in their normal schools. While they cited many examples of inspired teaching, they felt that the typical classroom was really no different from that in other schools. Though they found many teachers who were trying to accommodate themselves to the Gary concept and had faith in its workability, they also report that many felt confused and overburdened. Moreover, when evaluated against national standards of academic achievement (Courtis, 1919), the Gary students fared poorly. Even those who attended the Gary schools throughout their career did no better. Pupils did not seem to complete school in Gary any more than elsewhere and they were held back at about the same rate as in comparable cities. Dewey and Dewey (1915), however, claimed there was greater power of retention for Gary schools and that an unusually large number went on to college. While the Flexner and Bachman study is admirable in terms of its breadth and depth and its care in exposition, it does not speak of the community's feelings about the school, nor does it emphasize the school's students.

Flexner (1940) claimed that the Flexner-Bachman report effectively squelched interest in the Gary system. That estimate, as Cremin (1964) points out, is unquestionably wrong. Interest in the Gary system declined after the disastrous effort to introduce it into New York, and with the entrance of the United States into the First World War. The Gary School concept continued to be influential in American education well into the 1920's. Literally hundreds of communities adopted Gary ideas and modified aspects of their school system accordingly.

The criticisms of the Gary system are reported here to provide a balanced presentation. Moreover, the Flexner and Bachman report is an important document, presenting some of the problems in innovation and institutional change. The success of the Gary system is not the most important issue for our present purpose. Founded on a concept of the social and institutional causes of personal distress, the schools were designed to prevent or relieve social and mental health problems through a programmatic approach. The distress was to be countered by an enhancement of individuality and by an attempt to make school work real and relevant. Early visiting teachers were aware of the need for such a program and some of them worked toward it. The Gary concept, developed by an educator, shows the potential of the school as a model preventive mental health service. If the mental health professional wishes to prevent ills in society on a programmatic basis, then he also will have to consider developing and supporting ideas for institutional change.

8

the Chicago Juvenile Court and the Juvenile Psychopathic Institute

Urban poverty in the 1890's was accompanied by a high degree of familial and social disorganization, just as it is now. Then as now the people who appeared in the social agencies, the mental hospitals, and the jails were mostly the urban poor. The American conscience supported some form of care for dependent children in orphan homes, but under the influence of a conservative Social Darwinism, efforts to ameliorate the conditions of the poor were sporadic and inadequate. The dominant viewpoint of the 1870's is well expressed in the following paragraph from Herbert Spencer, the philosopher whose interpretation of Darwinism as a sign of continual progress made him a revered figure among American businessmen:

> Fostering the good for nothing at the expense of the good, is an extreme cruelty. It is a deliberate storing up of miseries for future generations. There is no greater curse to posterity than that of bequeathing them an increasing population of imbeciles, idlers and criminals. To aid the bad in multiplying, is, in effect, the same as maliciously providing for our descendants a multitude of enemies. It may be doubted whether the maudlin philanthropy which, looking only at direct mitigations, persistently ignores

indirect mischiefs, does not inflict a greater total of misery than the extremest selfishness inflicts (Spencer, 1873, p. 312).

origin of the Juvenile Court

Conservative Social Darwinism applied to children as well as adults; few special efforts were made to assist children in need, especially those who came into conflict with the law. Prior to 1899 only a few places treated children who committed crimes differently from adults. A few states authorized separate hearings for juveniles, but in most instances there were no special facilities for children who were arrested.

As early as 1824, a reformatory[1] was established in Elmira, New York, so that after conviction children would not have to be confined with adults, but in most states they were jailed with adult offenders, particularly while they awaited trial. If guilty the child was punished or placed on probation exactly as though he were an adult.

The Juvenile Court represented a marked change in conception, for not only was it established to deal with juveniles separately, but it was established with a sweeping mandate for child welfare. Furthermore, since it was a service which developed as a result of concerted community action, the Juvenile Court was a reflection of the humanitarianism that flowered in the last decades of the 19th century.

The first true Juvenile Court was established in Chicago July 1, 1899.[2] The regular courts in Chicago had treated juveniles separately from adults since 1861. The Juvenile Court was the result of the efforts

[1] Bordin (1964) describes one of the educative and rehabilitative reformatories of that day. Reformatories operated on the principles that productive labor, education, and a religious experience would effect the prisoner's reform. The approach of one matron, Emma Hall, is described in some detail by Bordin. Originally an educator, Emma Hall emphasized what her charges might become.

[2] Judge Ben Lindsey, whom we shall discuss in some detail in chapter 9, asserts a claim for precedence in establishing the Juvenile Court. Lindsey did not become a judge until 1901, but the law he used to create a Juvenile Court was passed in April, 1899, a few months before the establishment of the Chicago Juvenile Court (Lindsey, 1925).

of two groups, the Chicago Women's Club, under the leadership of Mrs. Lucy Flower, and Jane Addams' Hull House.

The women's clubs of that era were originally formed by upper-class women for their own cultural enrichment. Caught up in the moral and humanitarian mood of the 1890's, these clubs became a potent force for reform. They did not engage in direct charity but instead publicized the plight of the urban poor and lobbied for reform legislation. The General Federation of Women's Clubs, a national organization formed in 1890 and numbering a million members by 1912, championed a vigorous program of reform to assist women and children, to improve the schools and conditions under which they worked, to further consumer protection, and to beautify their communities (Hays, 1957). The Chicago Women's Club had had a Jail Committee as early as 1883. That committee called public attention to the fact that juveniles were treated as criminals and it proposed a separate Juvenile Court as early as 1892.

In 1898, the Illinois State Conference of Charities devoted its annual meeting to the subject of "The Children of the State." The conference, in which members of Chicago's Women's Club were well represented, agreed that there ought to be a children's court in Chicago. The committee which drafted the act included, among others, Mrs. Flower, president of the Chicago Women's Club, a judge who coped with the constitutional problems the act entailed, and the state representative who introduced the bill. The support of the Chicago Bar Association was enlisted. Mrs. Flower and her fellow clubwomen arranged for the judges of the various courts to be entertained at a luncheon at which the bill was announced. The Chicago Women's Club and other interested people further supported the Juvenile Court Bill by raising private funds to pay for the services of probation workers (Lathrop, 1925).

The women's clubs were actively involved with the operation of the court later on as well. Attached to the court was the detention home under the supervision of a member of the Juvenile Court Committee, which was composed of representatives from the various women's clubs. The Women's Club members made frequent, even daily visits to the detention home, to inspect its facilities and guarantee standards of cleanliness and care. A new courtroom was obtained because the women encouraged businessmen husbands and friends to lobby for them with the appropriate municipal officials. The Juvenile Court Committee participated in the selection of probation workers and interviewed and made recommendations for the appointment of the Juvenile Court judges. In the very earliest days of the court, two members of the Juvenile Court Committee regularly sat with the judge to advise or to assist in the disposition of cases (Bowen, 1925; Linn, 1935).

the settlement house and the non-professional probation worker

Hull House, a community action agency, played an important role in the development of the Juvenile Court as a helping agency. Jane Addams tells the story:

> From our earliest days, we saw many boys constantly arrested, and I had a number of enlightening experiences in the police station with an Irish lad whose mother upon her deathbed had begged me to "look after him." We were distressed by the gangs of very little boys who would sally forth with an enterprising leader in search of old brass and iron, sometimes breaking into empty houses for the sake of the faucets or lead pipe which they would sell for a good price to a junk dealer. With the money thus obtained they would buy cigarettes and beer or even candy, which could be conspicuously consumed in the alleys where they might enjoy the excitement of being seen and suspected by the "coppers." From the third year of Hull House, one of the residents held a semi-official position in the nearest police station, at least the sergeant agreed to give her provisional charge of every boy and girl under arrest for a trivial offense.
>
> Mrs. Stevens, who performed this work for several years, became the first probation officer of the Juvenile Court when it was established in Cook County in 1899. She was the sole probation officer at first, but at the time of her death, which occurred at Hull House in 1900, she was the senior officer of a corps of six. Her entire experience

had fitted her to deal wisely with wayward children. She had gone into a New England cotton mill at the age of thirteen,[3] where she had promptly lost the index finger of her right hand through "carelessness" she was told, and no one then seemed to understand that freedom from care was the prerogative of childhood. Later she became a member of the typographical union, retaining her "card" through all the later years of editorial work. As the Juvenile Court developed, the committee of public spirited citizens, who first supplied only Mrs. Stevens' salary, later maintained a corps of twenty-two such officers; several of these were Hull House residents who brought to the house for many years, a sad little procession of children struggling against all sorts of handicaps. When legislation was secured[4] which placed the probation officers upon the payroll of the county, it was a challenge to the efficiency of the civil service method of appointment to obtain by examination men and women fitted for this delicate human task. As one of five people asked by the civil service commission to conduct this

[3] Although it was fairly common for middle-class New England girls to work in factories in the early part of the 19th century, Mrs. Stevens, came from a working-class family and was a model "indigenous worker," to use today's term.

[4] The role and the power of the Chicago Women's Club is depicted by Mrs. Joseph T. Bowen, second president of the Chicago Juvenile Court Committee:

> We had at that time, a fine body of men and women who were most anxious for the success of the Court and for the good of the children, and we finally secured passage of a law which provided that probation officers be placed on the payroll of the county. I well remember how that law was passed, because it gave me a great feeling of uneasiness that it was so easy to accomplish. I happened to know at that time a noted Illinois politician. I asked him to my house and told him I wanted to get this law passed. The legislature was in session; he went to the telephone in my library, called up one of the bosses in the Senate and one in the House and said to each, "There is a bill, number so and so, which I want passed; see that it is done at once." One of the men whom he called evidently said, "What is there in it?" and the reply was, "There is nothing in it, but a woman I know wants it passed"—and it was passed. I thought with horror at the time, supposing it had been a bad bill, it would have been passed in exactly the same way (Bowen, 1925, p. 301).

Mrs. Bowen, a formidable Chicago aristocrat long associated with Hull House, was a driving force in developing the court, training probation workers, selecting the judges, and organizing the Juvenile Protective Association (Linn, 1935).

first examination for probation officers, I became convinced
that we were but at the beginning of the non-political
method of selecting public servants, but even still and
unbending as the examination may be, it is still our hope of
political salvation (Addams, 1910, pp. 323–325).

Placing the selection of probation workers under civil service
proved the kiss of death for the Juvenile Court in Chicago. The
public treasury proved niggardly in its support of probation workers
and the overloaded probation staff of the Chicago Court functioned
relatively inadequately. The record of children on probation in the
Chicago Court was quite poor compared to other cities (see
Chapter 9).

The quotation from Jane Addams indicates that she debated the
relative costs and benefits of civil service for selecting probation
officers. Judge Lindsey, William Healy, and many others responsible
for the development and operation of the early court recognized
that the personal qualifications of probation officers were vital
factors determining whether or not the individual functioned effectively
with children as a probation officer. Mrs. Bowen states the case:

I think the first probation officer was Mrs. Alzina Stevens,
perhaps the best example of what a probation officer should
be. Her great desire was to be of use to her fellow men.
Her love of children was great; her singleness of purpose
and strength of character so remarkable that she exerted
a great influence over the children committed to her charge.
I find among some old papers the following concerning the
duties of probation officers: "They must be men and women
of many sides, endowed with the strength of a Samson and
the delicacy of an Ariel. They must be tactful, skillful, firm
and patient. They must know how to proceed with wisdom
and intelligence and must be endowed with that rare virtue
—common sense." These qualities would seem to be needed
just as much today as they were twenty-five years ago
(Bowen, 1925, pp. 299–300).

The "unbending" civil service examination did not attempt to
select people who had the necessary personal qualifications to do the

job. Why didn't the Juvenile Court seek more people like Mrs. Stevens?

Lincoln Steffens' muckraking classic, *Shame of the Cities* (1904), described political corruption rampant in cities across the United States. Political bosses maintained their control in part through patronage appointments to municipal agencies. Municipal reformers were in favor of a civil service system as a means of curbing the power of the ward bosses. That the tactic was effective can be seen in Tammany boss Plunkitt's complaints that the civil service was a curse upon mankind, undermining the loyalty of one man to another and destroying the patriotic feeling which brought good Americans out to Fourth of July picnics and political orations (Riordan, 1905).

Municipal reformers, to be consistent with their principles, had to support civil service appointments for probation workers, even though then as now, the objective civil service test could not measure personality qualifications. While those who operated the court might have been able intuitively to select workers with the necessary traits, this method of selection would have laid them open to charges of inconsistency and of operating their own patronage system. Here is an excellent example of how larger issues in the society influence the course of development of a helping service in ways which may have nothing to do with the needs of the service.

the Juvenile Court as a helping agency

The Juvenile Court is not generally thought of as a helping agency, but the legal principle under which it was established had enormous significance for the concept that child welfare was indeed the responsibility of the state. The legal principle not only took the child's case out of the criminal courts, but it established that the court was to deal with the children under its power of *parens patriae* and in chancery or civil jurisdiction.

The significance of this change is discussed by Judge Julian Mack, first judge of the Chicago Juvenile Court. Chancery procedure, he points out, established

> the conception that a child that broke the law was to be
> dealt with by the state, as a wise parent would deal with a

wayward child. . . . That is the conception that the State is
the higher parent; that it has an obligation, not merely
a right but an obligation, toward its children; and that is a
specific obligation to step in when the natural parent, either
through viciousness or inability, fails so to deal with the
child that it no longer goes along the right path that leads
to good sound, adult citizenship. . . . The State always
stepped in when there was property involved, took charge
of the property and appointed a guardian, and when it
appointed a guardian for the property, it appointed a
guardian of the person of the child. But until the Juvenile
Court law was enacted, nobody seemed to think of the possibility of extending this principle of the whole parenthood
of the state, the ultimate parenthood of the State towards
its little ones. No one before that seemed to think that the
State ought to be and ought to act as the wise parent or the
natural parent, or to undertake successfully to guide the
child along the right way (Mack, 1925, pp. 311–312).

The statutes under which the Juvenile Courts were established
included exceedingly broad definitions of delinquency, in keeping with
the new concept. A complaint against a child in the Juvenile Court
is not an indictment; it is usually called a "petition in behalf of the
child." According to Sutherland and Cressey (1960), the precise
definition of delinquency is rarely established in Juvenile Court law.
Jurisdiction is established over those whose "occupation, behavior,
environment or associations are injurious to his welfare," and over
those who violate any state law or municipal ordinance. The Colorado
statute, for example, included children who were "vicious, incorrigible,
or immoral in conduct," who were "habitually truant" (an offense
created by the passage of compulsory school attendance laws), or who
were deemed to be "disorderly persons."

The conception underlying the Juvenile Court law, in effect, gave
the Juvenile Court full responsibility for child guidance and child
welfare. The Juvenile Court statutes not only defined delinquency for
the mental health professions, but they also established the court as the
institution which has responsibility for the care and amelioration of a

variety of interpersonal and emotional difficulties of childhood.[5] It is this concept which makes it understandable that Healy's clinic was later established as part of the Juvenile Court.

probation and prevention

In the early days of the Chicago Court, the probation workers were supported by private, not public funds. Associated with the court was the Juvenile Protective Association, whose membership consisted of the twenty-two privately supported probation workers, many of whom were also settlement house workers, and the executive committee of the citizens' group which financed them. The Juvenile Protective Association thought in preventive terms. They identified conditions in the city which adversely affected the lives of children and young people and acted to correct these conditions. The association worked with the Druggist's Association to induce its members to stop selling indecent postcards; with the Saloon Keeper's Association to stop selling liquor to minors; with the Grocer's Association to stop tobacco sales to minors; with department store managers to supply matrons to help reduce shoplifting; with watchmen in the railroad yards to get them to report boys to the association instead of arresting them for trespassing; with theater owners to provide wholesome entertainment; and with film makers to develop educational materials which presented information about health and morals entertainingly and instructively.[6] The association worked to have social centers opened, to turn unused buildings into recreation centers, to turn lots into gardens, to organize hiking parties, to develop bathing beaches, and to open public schools for social purposes. It was partly through the efforts of the Association that Healy's clinic was initiated.

[5] In 1966, the Supreme Court ruled that the Juvenile Courts must extend the full protection of due process to children. While admirable from the point of view of individual rights, we believe Justice Fortas' decision did not reflect sufficient indignation about the inadequate treatment rendered children by a governmental institution charged with their care and not their punishment.

[6] Whatever one might think of the desirability of these measures, it is to be noted the members worked to correct social conditions they believed contributed to the development of delinquency while they worked with the individual delinquent. It is likely that later civil service probation workers would not see preventive, pro-

origin of the Juvenile Psychopathic Institute

The probation work of the Juvenile Protective Association was largely carried out with the philosophy that the children who came before the court were not bad, but in need of satisfying, purposeful activities. It was felt that education and appropriate activities would prevent further difficulty. However, the court workers quickly encountered many cases which defied such simple understanding and treatment. For example, a seven-year-old cherub with long curls down his back, who was in the detention home associated with the court, poured kerosene over all the beds and set fire to them. There were children who repeatedly stole, lied, or who committed sexual offenses for reasons which remained obscure.

Encountering these cases, the Juvenile Protective Association, stimulated by an active member, Mrs. Ethel S. Dummer, called for scientific research into the causes of such behavior.[7] Mrs. Dummer promised financial support for such a project for five years. A committee chaired by Julia Lathrop, a Hull House Settlement worker, met at Hull House to select a man for the job. The man who was selected, with recommendations by James R. Angell, William James, and Adolph Meyer, was William Healy.

Healy, who was born in England, had studied psychology with William James at Harvard. Healy was at Harvard when Adolph Meyer was at the nearby Worcester State Hospital. Meyer had written about child psychiatry from 1895 onward and, given Healy's interest in pediatric neurology, it is likely they were in contact with each other. In the *Individual Delinquent* (Healy, 1915), Healy credits his approach to the case history to Adolph Meyer. Healy obtained his M.D. degree at Rush Medical School in Chicago in 1900. His psychiatric training

---

grammatic work as part of their job. In fact, independent community action by probation workers would probably be barred in most cities. The difference in approach in contemporary courts reflects, in part, the problem of the institutionalization and the professionalization of innovation.

[7] John Dewey's influence, however indirect, is worth noting in this context. Because of Dewey, the Chicago public schools had established a Child Study Department to help with children's problems. His interest, and the interest of men such as Angell, Mead, and Tufts, established a precedent in Chicago for the scientific study of the real problems of the day (Addams, 1929).

seems to have consisted of experience as assistant physician at the Wisconsin State Hospital from 1900 to 1901 and a post-graduate year in Vienna, Berlin, and London from 1906–1907. No convenient record indicates whether Healy had any contact with the early psychoanalytic groups. However, his interest in psychoanalysis and its methods was apparent in his first large report on his work with the Chicago Court, *The Individual Delinquent* (Healy, 1915).

Healy practiced in Chicago as a neurologist and developed a reputation for his ability to treat children, some of whom had been referred to him by the Juvenile Court. His public statements against punitive handling of children in the home and the court brought him to the attention of the Juvenile Protective Association. The association had discovered there were many puzzling cases which could be neither understood nor helped by their approach. They were also concerned that the Juvenile Court judge had to make decisions about the disposition of children without adequate knowledge. The judge said he was "often in a fog" about given cases and that he would welcome any help he might receive from the careful study of individual cases.

Healy decided to establish a research project into the causes of delinquency, coupled with a clinic to treat children's behavior problems. Before establishing his clinic, he toured the country and found that, with the exception of Witmer's clinic and Goddard's laboratory at Vineland, no facilities then in existence employed psychological examination with physical examination in the diagnostic study of children. Healy named his clinic the Juvenile Psychopathic Institute because of prevalent psychiatric opinion that serious anti-social behavior implied serious psychopathology. This theoretical viewpoint was based on very little firsthand study and it was a view Healy soon discovered to be incorrect.

The Juvenile Psychopathic Institute was organized in March, 1909, with a five-year endowment from Mrs. Ethel S. Dummer.[8] Healy's institute had the benefit of a distinguished advisory council with James R. Angell, George H. Mead, and Adolph Meyer among the members.

[8] The influence of the source of funds on the work done may be surmised from Mrs. Dummer's comments. Healy's discussion of the unconscious and his attempts to help by methods of psychotherapy apparently elicited criticism from the local intellectual community. "Some Juvenile Protective Association members wanted a committee to pass on Healy's findings before publication. Holding the purse strings, I insisted his results were his own and he was free to publish as he pleased. This caused a break with the Association" (Dummer, 1948, p. 10).

Jane Addams and Julia Lathrop, later Chief of the Children's Bureau in Washington, were members of the executive committee. John Wigmore, the dean of Northwestern's law school and a member of the advisory council, was instrumental in bringing Healy's work to the attention of the law schools.

The Juvenile Psychopathic Institute did not develop as an isolated entity; it was a part of the reform movement of the time and clearly influenced in its direction and operation by the predominant intellectual views. For example, although Healy does not cite George Herbert Mead or other early sociologists in the Chicago School of Social Sciences, his discussion of the psychology of the delinquent in relation to the problem and its treatment seems to contain a large element of the period's sociological thought (Healy, 1925). However, his focus on the characteristics of the individual, coming near the end of the period of reform, seems to be a portent of the post-war period.

Healy's clinic

In April of 1909, Healy, psychologist Grace Fernald, and a secretary constituted the first staff of the clinic. The clinic was housed within the detention home in the same building where the daily sessions of the Juvenile Court were held. Augusta F. Bronner, who was to become a long-time associate of Healy's and eventually his wife, joined the clinic in 1913. Bronner had been Thorndike's assistant at Teachers' College, Columbia University, and she brought a strong interest in educational problems as they related to delinquency.

In the first years of the clinic the profession of psychiatric social work did not exist. Social histories and the treatment of families were the responsibility of social workers from other agencies and of well-trained probation workers. Professional psychiatric social work did not come to the Juvenile Psychopathic Institute until after 1917. By that time, Dr. Herman Adler had succeeded Healy, who had left to establish the Judge Baker Guidance Center in Boston.

Healy's task was to study the individual delinquent. He devised a highly detailed, exceedingly thorough examination. The full examination included a family history; a developmental history; a history of the social environment; a history of mental and moral development, including school history, friends, interests, occupational history, bad habits; and a history of the individual's contacts with law enforcement agencies or institutions. A complete medical examination from psychiatric and neurological standpoints was conducted and anthropometric and psychological studies were completed. For purposes of the psychological study Healy and Bronner devised a number of performance tests of their own. (In this, they were apparently advised by Angell, then chairman of the department of psychology at the University of Chicago.) The tests, the examinations, and their purposes were discussed in detail in *The Individual Delinquent*. It is of considerable interest to see how Healy anticipated later psychological studies of delinquency in the tests he devised and the traits he chose to study.

Healy kept a careful record of delinquencies committed by each subject and careful follow-up records. His data included a diagnostic and prognostic summary and an attempt to judge, insofar as he could, the most important causes in the case. His record forms were devised by Mr. Dummer, a business executive. There are probably few child guidance centers of the present day which offer as complete a diagnostic work-up as did Healy or Witmer in those early days.

relationship to the court

Healy was interested in studying delinquency, but on a clinical level he was also performing a service. For some time he sat in on the daily sessions of the Juvenile Court and was asked his opinion as cases came up. He soon realized that he had little more basis than the judge to offer an opinion on a child he had not studied, so he abandoned the practice. It became his job to make recommendations to the court and the probation workers for the treatment or the disposition of various cases, but only after a thorough study of the child. From comments he makes (Healy & Bronner, 1926; Healy & Bronner, 1948), it is clear that the courts did not always follow his recommendations, despite their request for his services.

There were a variety of dispositional alternatives, although resources were indeed slim at that time in Chicago. First, a child might be placed on probation under the supervision of a probation officer. In various places Healy commented on how the differences in personality between probation workers influenced their effectiveness with children. Secondly, he might be placed in a foster home, often with a family on a farm, or, as Healy put it, "placed in country life." A third possible disposition was commitment to a correctional institution or to an institution for dependent children.

These institutions had widely varying characteristics and the one chosen could make a considerable difference in the life of a child. The Chicago Parental School was maintained by the Board of Education. Children of school age were committed there by the court for an average stay of five months. The school was organized on the cottage plan, offered regular school subjects, manual training, and excellent recreational facilities. A second short-term institution, abandoned soon after Healy's association with the court, was the John Worthy School, noted for its exceedingly strict disciplinary control. A third institution was the State Training School, serving the state of Illinois. Its chief drawback was the parole system, which employed only one officer for the entire state. In addition there were a number of church-related or privately owned institutions for dependent children which offered residential care, general education, and shop work. Finally, there were a small number of institutions for the care and training of girls.

Healy viewed the problem of placement as an empirical question requiring careful research. He made recommendations for disposition on the basis of intensive studies and as a scientist, he was concerned with following-up the children in their different settings. The follow-up reports of cases studied in Boston reflects the care and attention to detail Healy displayed in his clinical and research work (Healy & Bronner, 1926).

views on therapy—programmatic approaches

Although Healy's reputation is based on his application of psychotherapeutic methods and psychoanalytic concepts to delinquency, he was extraordinarily broad in his viewpoint toward treatment. He did not arbitrarily exclude any form of intervention which might produce a desirable behavioral change. Although chary about the efficacy of a punitive approach, he indicated his understanding that a judicial system could not function without punishment. He even wrote of some cases benefited by exposure to harsh treatment in an institutional setting. His brief discussion of religious education and treatment reveals his openmindedness and his scientific acumen.

Healy was fully aware of the necessity for programmatic approaches. He argued that the availability and quality of resources for recreation, education, foster home placement, and other child welfare measures had a vital relationship to the causes and treatment of delinquency. Evidently difficulties with cooperation between services already existed, for he also recommended development of a method to coordinate services. An organization to monitor the social conditions causing delinquent conduct was a part of the total program he recommended.

The failures to heed the recommendations of early pioneers reflect, we believe, not the unsoundness of their recommendations, but the fact that helping services are determined by factors beyond current theories of personality and psychopathology. The continued difficulties in coordinating social agencies fifty years later, to the detriment of individuals in need of help (Sarason, et al., 1966), illustrates that the recognition alone of the problem is insufficient to correct it. Similarly, the experiences of earlier workers in delinquency and their emphasis on the social and environmental aspects of delinquency was simply ignored by later workers who tried to develop psychotherapeutic approaches. It is in the 1960's that once again we see renewed attention to the social conditions which cause delinquency and renewed attention to programmatic approaches to the problem.

A full program would also take into account the characteristics of the court and the police, for Healy felt that the way the police handled an offender and the way the courts treated an offender affected what happened to him later. In some cases Healy sensed that an element of sport entered the delinquent's relationship with the police; the delinquent risked penalty against the possibility he could escape detection. Healy implies that some modification of the relationship between the law enforcing agencies and the individual might have a beneficial effect not only in the rehabilitation of a given individual but also in the prevention of delinquent acts.

A full program would involve efforts to change public attitudes toward crime and the criminal. Healy felt that in many groups the delinquent and the criminal were held up as culture heroes and that crime was viewed as a form of adventure. This comment, found in a book written in 1926 (Healy & Bronner, 1926), may reflect the ethos of the "Roaring Twenties."

psychotherapeutic methods

Environmental manipulation, with the help of church, school, and social agencies, was one part of his treatment of children. In addition, Healy worked psychotherapeutically with individuals and also in what he called the reeducation of families. Unfortunately, the literature we have been able to find does not contain a good description of his specific approach to individuals and to families. Healy's writings carefully describe the characteristics of individuals and delinquent populations. He produced much case material from the delinquent's "Own Story," but left us little that helps us to understand his conduct of interviews. In the material that follows, we have had to take bits and pieces from his writings in order to illustrate his methods of working. He himself criticized *The Individual Delinquent* because it contains an insufficient discussion of treatment.

Although he debated with himself whether the physician or the psychologist is best equipped to handle the problems which arise, he believed the psychologist's approach of first importance:

The only attitude to be assumed with much profit is that of shrewd but sympathetic inquiry into an unsolved problem. We have insisted that the examiner should have no special nose for the pathological and should be willing to survey all the facts, and to be guided in his conclusions by no special bias. The question for him must be: What is the cause in this person or in his experience and how can it be altered?

Often I have stated the following fact, which has become increasingly apparent to me. Just as soon as the offender and his relative realize there is someone who takes the attitude of the friendly family physician, to whom they can go with their secret troubles, the case frequently undergoes the most remarkable transformation from the fighting aspect actually seen in the court room or while the interested ones are in contact with the police or other authorities of the law.

The opening of the interview with some such friendly and reasonable statement as the following has been found in itself to have a rationalizing effect. One may say: "Well, you people do seem to have a difficult affair on your hands with this boy. Let's sit down and talk it all over, and study it out together—how it all began and what's going to happen. I'm at your service. Did you ever think it all out carefully?" (Healy, 1915, pp. 36–37).

The timing of the interviews is an important issue. Healy describes the "golden moment" for intervention during a period of crisis and the value of being a part of the court:

The offender must approach you willingly before you can do anything for him. Now when will he exhibit this willingness? Certainly not when he is "on the outs" and feeling it quite unlikely that he will recommit offenses or at least be caught again. No, the golden moment is when he feels himself to be a problem, and his relatives feel it, and all want a promising solution of the difficulty. It is after he has been caught, and while he is either detained or on probation, and has not already been sentenced that is the best time of all for inquiry. Then parents will come many miles in search of a solution, not by any means always desiring the softest outcomes for the offender. Then the offender will himself strive hardest to achieve with the "doctor" some fundamental explanation of the causes of his delinquent tendencies (pp. 40–41).

The problem of initial resistance was handled in the following manner:

Over and over from relatives and others we have heard of the difficulty in getting their problem individual to come

and see us. It seems to be hard to get it understood that
because there is delinquency there must be need of study.
The answer is given, "There is nothing the matter with me.
I know what I'm doing," so it comes about that a collateral
explanation is offered. "We want you to go to see the doctor
to find out if you are healthy," or, "We want to find out
what you are best fitted for." This latter explanation indeed
makes a truthful form of entrance that we have come to use
most frequently as offering the chance of developing the
greatest amount of interest. The question of vocational
diagnosis is really part of almost every young person's
thoughts, however crudely apperceived. . . . In all this tact
is of greatest service and one learns to develop an elastic
method which best of all subserves scientific as well as
practical interests (pp. 45–46).

Healy preferred to use a series rather than a single interview
because he recognized that the positive and negative conclusions based
on a single interview were likely to be erroneous. He preferred to
deal with the patient and his relatives one at a time for he felt that in
private interviews he discovered friction in the household more
effectively, and that in any event people preferred to be alone with
their physicians when telling their troubles.

Apparently he approached his cases with great openness and
directness, despite what one might think from his emphasis on an
approach through vocational interests. In dealing with pathological
lying, for example, he recommends direct confrontation.

In discussing treatment great emphasis should be placed
upon the primary necessity for directly meeting the pathological liar upon the level of the moral failures and making
it plain that these are known and understood. It is very
certain that frequently this type of prevaricator has very
little conception of the social antagonism which his habit
arouses. . . . When it comes to specific details of treatment,
these must be educational, alterative and constructive. In
cases 1 and 3 under treatment we know that when the lying
was discovered or suspected the individual was at once
checked up and made to go over the ground and state the

real facts. The pathological liar ordinarily reacts to the accusation of lying by prevaricating again in self-defense, but when with the therapeutist there has been the understanding that the tendency to lying is a habit which it is necessary to break, the barricade of self-defense may not be thrown up (Healy & Healy, 1926, pp. 273–274).

Healy practiced psychoanalysis himself, and with others wrote an important textbook on psychoanalysis (Healy, Bronner, & Bowers, 1931). It is instructive to note that he was not precious about brief psychotherapies, as many were later during the 1950's and 1960's (Healy, 1915, p. 119). Rather, he felt brief therapeutic interviews were effective:

With these [few cases], however, there were some startlingly good results which proved much to us particularly when in the interview some youngster recalled a traumatic episode and verbalized the attendant and often continuing emotional upset. . . . There were failures, perhaps due to not using more skilled techniques or perhaps to not being able to alter reality situations, but there is no gainsaying the fact that comparatively few interviews involving no deeply penetrating interpretations did work wonders in some cases of serious misconduct, and still do (Healy & Bronner, 1948, p. 29).

Although enthusiastic about the possibilities inherent in psychoanalysis, Healy was also acutely sensitive to the limitations of a solely psychoanalytic approach.

The therapeutic effects of the application of the psychoanalytic method to the study of offenders prove in some instances nothing short of brilliant. . . .

By merely showing to the subject, through hauling up the contents of his own mental reservoirs, what his failure is based on may not prove sufficient, if environmental or physical conditions which serve as two of the three instigating causes, are still irritating as of old. Various reasons will readily suggest why this should be so. Habits and thoughts

and tendencies of years' standing are not to be lightly overcome if nothing but added knowledge is to stand up against
them. Re-education and helpful new interests from the outside are also frequently necessary. For energies which previously found outlet in socially undesirable behavior, "sub-
stitution" must be made possible by discovery of a junction
point where now by conscious volition, shunting on to
another track can take place (Healy, 1915, pp. 120–121).

child guidance—work with parents

Healy worked in child guidance, that is, he worked with the parents
of the children he saw. He preferred to work with both the children and
the parents himself, rather than have one person see the parent
and another the child, as is frequent in later child guidance practice.
While he was interested in the parent's "Own Story," too, and while
he recognized the role of parental friction and discord in producing
mental conflict and delinquency, he did not seem to blame the parents.
Sometimes he worked with parents to help them express a particular
personal problem, but he treated parents as intelligent persons who
could, if given sufficient direction, take hold and help solve the
problems.

For example, one case was that of a ten-year-old girl who had
engaged in petty stealing and had been expelled from two schools.
Healy discovered the child was obsessed with sexual thoughts. He
advised the mother to give her child sexual information and suggested
measures to keep her busy at school and at home.

In another case, that of a sixteen-year-old boy who had run away
from home, and who had at various times forged his father's name to
get money, Healy made specific recommendations for treatment:

In this case a definite tendency to delinquency was under
consideration, a tendency that had not been modified by

admonitions or threats. The outlook now, with understanding of beginnings, was altogether different. The coffee and smoking should be stopped, the evening reading, which had been somewhat opposed, should be allowed at home, but above all there must be modification of parental behavior. The scolding, even though justified, and especially the speaking of the boy behind his back, should be abandoned. The mediation which our discoveries led us to offer, was well received, and the father's negotiations for placing the boy in a reformatory situation were broken off. For the six months elapsed since we saw this case, the report is that there has been an entire change of conduct (Healy, 1915, p. 397).

the necessity for follow-up

For Healy, the essence of treatment (and of research) was the follow-up:

As one makes more and more studies of the formative period of life, and watches cases go on to success or failure, one sees clearly that a great feature of treatment is the careful carrying over of offenders through the period of adolescent instability. A little touch here and a little touch there to the young individual is not sufficient; there must be that prolonged studying of the case that offers the best chance of forfending the growth of delinquent tendencies. . . .

A very weak point in practically all social and moral therapy is the lack of follow-up work. Criticism may be extended to parents who have no patience to deal systematically with a problem child, to court admonitions which imply the ability of human nature to change itself in a trice, to public administration which sends back old offenders from institutions to an environment where they are almost sure to fail again (Healy, 1915, p. 178).

residential treatment

In the early days, Healy did not operate a residential treatment center or a correctional institution, but he studied and acted as consultant for many such institutions. In 1915, Healy and Bronner wrote an outline for a model correctional institution, based not only upon first-hand observation, but also upon their diagnostic and follow-up studies of individuals treated in various institutions. Portions of that outline are reproduced here, both because the program of milieu therapy is so modern in tone, and because it reflects the educative approach so fully.

After discussing goals (to fit the individual to cope with all phases of an ordinary social environment), the physical equipment, the selection of staff ("The selection of working personnel is the most important single consideration. The influence of a man or woman of good understanding upon youthful delinquents, whenever in contact with them, is not to be overvalued"), and the urgent need for adequate follow-up after release, Healy and Bronner go on to lay out the treatment program for an institution to serve delinquent children.

> Treatment in general: Before discussing specific phases of treatment, its general moods and aims should be taken up.
>
> (a) The entire institutional life should be adjusted with the ideal that it is treatment, that it is educational, and all to the end that the delinquent shall be better fitted to meet an outside environment.
>
> (b) This requires high individualization. One of the arguments against the advisability of a set system is found in the successes which are actually obtained by a rational and understanding approach to the problem of the individual. Both education and work must be adapted to the individual needs.
>
> (c) Three things to avoid are any kind of deceit, the show of pedantry, and any demonstration of irrationality. It is most desirous to make the individual rational and honest, and this can only be done by showing a good example in these respects.[9]

[9] Compare this point with Redl and Wineman's (1951) discussion of the sensitivity of delinquent children to corruption or pretense in the staff.

(d) The method should be elastic in all ways, particularly in institutions for girls, where allowance must be made for outbreaks and explosions of pent-up emotions and energies, either occasional or periodic.[10] Of course, physical fluctuations must be allowed for.

(e) Punishments: These must be highly individualized according to personalities involved. There is no doubt that stimulus to doing better is more apt to result from the promise of rewards than the administering of penalties. There must be goals toward which the delinquent is to work as the reward of good behavior. With constructive treatment the problems of discipline largely tend to disappear. It should be remembered that coercion and punishment by inflicting pain are the lowest levels of control.

(f) Above all things, mental vacuities, either on week days or Sundays, must be prevented. "The empty mind is the devil's workshop." There should be abundant opportunity for good conversational reactions. This may be as important as formal instruction, and always the mental life should be the first and foremost consideration.

(g) The whole institutional equipment should be used with the sole idea of its social and moral worth.

(h) General social and educational life should include the planning of service and of rendering helpfulness to others in the institution. Cultivation of this is worth much, and from it can be built up larger ideas of social relationships. Perhaps the best way to avoid jealousies is to inculcate the idea of service, one to the other in the institution.[11]

(i) Intimate social life: One of the best helps toward a better life is an understanding friend and advisor with

[10] See Bordin's (1964) description of such periodic outbursts as taken from Emma Hall's diary of her experiences in the Michigan Reform School for Girls in the early 1800's.

[11] The concept of having an institutional ethos promoted actively by the staff should be compared with the development of a delinquent subculture in institutions where the professional staff function primarily as psychotherapists and where they relinquish responsibility for day-by-day programming to an untrained home staff. Polsky's book, *Cottage Six* (1962), describes the development and operation of such a subculture in one residential treatment center.

whom the cause and the help for trouble may be discussed.[12]

(j) In considering treatment in general it must not be thought that building up is always the point, or that positive habits are the only good; the inhibitions of bad impulses must be also considered. In some cases excessive physical vigor, or obstinancy of will, make special forms of modification necessary.

Dress: A moot question is over the dress of the institutional inmates. One point stands out clearly proven; namely, that any self-expression that is practicable in this matter should be cultivated.

Work: The arrangement of work to be done by the inmates has its economic and also its social and moral values. The immediate economies must not conflict with the aims of the institution. If the work has a deteriorating effect, or is interfering with treatment, it should be done by outsiders. But this does not mean that difficult or even so-called menial work should be neglected. The idea of duty on the part of the spelling[13] may be cultivated, although perhaps with difficulty in early adolescence, through the understanding that the institution ought to be largely self-sustaining. Work of all kinds is done, chiefly for common welfare. If it is merely assigned as a matter of routine or punishment without this feeling, work is apt to be detrimental and cause a grudge.

Very much of housework and other work can be done in the spirit of scientific training. There may be attention to skill and success in many household occupations. It must be shrewdly recognized that there may be great benefits accruing to selected individuals through their engaging in hard labor, either physical or mental, or both.

Religion: Religious training would be out of place to discuss here. In general, we may say that religious training which takes the individual as one of a group and does not

---

[12] This is almost the entire reference to the place of psychotherapy or counseling in the residential center.

[13] Healy and Bronner use the term "spelling" to mean a work shift. Their sensitivity to the possible exploitation of youth in correctional institutions bears underlining.

meet special problems is not apt to get results. Then it must be remembered, in all common sense, that natures differ greatly. The religious appeal is very strong in some, and others are oblivious to it (pp. 307–309).

Much of the remainder of the outline is a detailed curriculum for a school program. Dewey's influence is not acknowledged in the article, but the influence of progressive education is seen in the author's emphasis that in each instance subject matter was to be taught in a manner relevant to the adolescent's life situation and to therapeutic goals. Thus, subject matter might center around the female's role in the home and the male's role in the working world. There would be a great deal of emphasis on vocational possibilities and upon life in the community. The curriculum would include work on local political organizations, social welfare agencies, and educational and recreational resources in the community. All of these items in the curriculum reflected the goals of educational reformers (Cremin, 1964).

Healy and Bronner point out that a standard curriculum would have little utility for adolescents with a great deal of living experience and little formal educational training. They argue that any standard reading series would be useless. Reading materials should be of interest and have concrete applicability to the immediate life situation in order to emphasize the enjoyment and utility of reading. Music, art, and dramatics would also be part of the curriculum, with an emphasis upon participation and "spontaneous and joyful expression."[14] Dramatic performances were seen as opportunities to develop cooperative effort and practical skills in making costumes and in designing and building stage sets.

Arithmetic, writing, and spelling should emphasize what is actually needed and used in everyday life. For example, instruction in arithmetic should emphasize application to keeping household and other accounts.

Language should be taught specifically for the purpose of developing powers of expression and for the exchange of opinions. Healy and Bronner suggest that verbal expression be encouraged through "free

[14] In one residential treatment institution, we observed a music teacher who painfully persisted in trying to teach musical notation to a group of bored, resisting adolescents. On several occasions when he was absent, a substitute teacher brought in a guitar and taught folk songs to the same group, who became lively, interested, and presented no discipline problems at all.

and frank discussion of actual living problems that arise daily or that have arisen in the past.[15] There should be no specified period for this, but it should be done as the occasion arises" (p. 311).

Physical education is viewed as an opportunity not only for exercise, but for social participation, for the opportunity to develop cooperative effort, team spirit, and self-discipline.

Healy and Bronner suggest that a variety of special educational resources be available, but they are explicit that the formation of special classes to meet individual needs is undesirable. They also emphasize the consulting role of the psychiatrist or psychologist in the educational process.

> No one of these [special educational or therapeutic programs] necessitates the withdrawal from the ordinary classroom during the whole day or the formation of special classes. The special teacher should give daily such time as the individual case requires in the special field, whereas other work can be carried on in the regular classroom. The cooperation between teacher and diagnostician should be particularly close in these cases (p. 315).

Their outline contains a brief comment on the possibilities for self-government. Healy and Bronner are in favor of some form of self-government, but they point out that external control by staff is still necessary. One wonders whether Healy and Bronner had some opportunity to observe a development such as is described in William Golding's novel, *Lord of the Flies*, where unsocialized children legitimized authority by physical strength.

The outline, surprisingly complete and modern in its presentation, stresses the educative, therapeutic, and rehabilitative potential of every aspect of the institutional setting. The tone of the institution and the importance of all staff members as therapeutic agents are points of emphasis, as are the relevance of the curriculum to the needs and interests of the adolescent. Healy and Bronner realize that there will always be problems in management. In too many institutional settings, the staff seem to respond with the expectation that no management

---

[15] Compare with the contemporary emphasis on patient-staff ward conferences which take place in many milieu-therapy-oriented institutions.

problems should arise, and if they do, they are seen as staff failures, rather than as expected incidents or therapeutic opportunities.

The emphasis on an educative approach is also instructive in that psychopathological manifestations are not emphasized. There is no indication that Healy and Bronner found it necessary to obtain an admission of illness as a prerequisite to receiving help. The individual is placed in a situation in which the staff, the peer group, and the program itself are the therapeutic or change agents and it is assumed that the appropriate responses such stimuli elicit will result in behavioral change. Healy and Bronner recognize that in some instances, "delinquencies which arise on the basis of obsessive mental imagery" will require "special counteractive aids," but even these are integrated within the special educational environment. They emphasize a living through in a structured environment rather than a working through on a verbal-conceptual basis in a psychotherapeutic relationship. Although Healy practiced psychotherapy, he saw it as having a special place in the program. He clearly recognized there were other means of helping.

Healy and Bronner anticipated criticism of their program. The outline closes with the following paragraph:

> We would firmly contend that the above scheme is not Utopian; it is thoroughly practicable where a group of intelligent and well trained workers can be gathered in an institution. The basis of our survey of the subject is simply, as we have said, experiences with the needs of delinquents, and successes and failures of treatment. If our ideas of constructive efforts appear complex and difficult, it must be remembered that they are not any more so than the details of education and home life in any well conducted school and family. As for ultimate values accruing from such efforts—well, we are told that in Heaven there is much rejoicing over even one delinquent saved (p. 316).

summary

The Juvenile Court was an instrument and a product of the reform movement which flourished at the turn of the century. The problem

of delinquency was prominent because of the issues created by urbanization, industrialization, and poverty with its attendant social and
familial disorganization. In concept, the court's responsibility changed
from determining guilt and setting punishment to rehabilitating and
guiding "as a wise parent would guide a wayward child." The social
action and legal principles underlying the establishment of the Juvenile
Court made it explicit that the community was responsible for the
welfare of all in the community. The early Juvenile Courts, not only
in Chicago but throughout the country, were firmly embedded in the
community, with lay people taking a great deal of responsibility for
the court's work. In Chicago, volunteer organizations and a settlement
house which was part of the community worked to establish the court.
What we now call the "power structure" was instrumental in its growth
and development and in its early operation. Lindsey's Denver Court,
as we shall see in the next chapter, Hoffman's Cincinnati Court, and
Stubbs' Indianapolis Court were all closely tied in with their communities. In Philadelphia the early probation workers were supported
by the churches and synagogues, mothers' clubs, the settlement
houses, and private philanthropy (International Prison Commission,
1904). Healy's clinic developed as a result of community initiative,
and it too was integrated into the work of the court. Consciously or
not, those who planned this early clinical service understood the value
of a strategic location near the manifestation of the problem. The
clinical service in the court did not wait passively for the child or
the family in need to seek out the helping agency.

Healy's clinical methods and his thinking about delinquency are
worthy of note. Although he was quite familiar with the dynamic
concepts of psychoanalysis, he adopted a highly flexible approach in
his thinking and methods, recognizing the importance of creating
personality change by permitting the individual to live out his problems
in a new environment. Healy's psychodynamic approach, his willingness
to use psychological methods, his departure from seeking merely to
establish a diagnosis, and even his willingness to work in the community were remarkable innovations, considering the hospital psychiatry of his day. However, running throughout all of his therapeutic
work is an emphasis on what the person might become and a lesser
emphasis on what his psychopathology is. Healy says, ". . . the examiner
should have no special nose for the pathological. . . . The question for
him must be what is the cause in this person or in his experience and

how can it be altered?" In this view, at this time, he seemed to share the mood and attitude of the social and political reformers, who also had boundless faith in every man's potential, if only every man was provided the proper conditions to fulfill his potential.

In the following chapter, we shall present the work of a remarkable man of the same era, Judge Ben B. Lindsey of the Denver Juvenile Court. Lindsey, a lawyer by profession, a politician by nature, and a reformer by conviction, was a psychological and social therapist of immense skill. In the Denver Court of the early 1900's we find two principles, of embeddedness in the community, and faith that each man contains the spark of the divine, combined with unusual power, beauty, and effectiveness.

9

Judge Ben Lindsey
and the Denver Juvenile Court:
an institution of human relations

Am I a judge now? I AM NOT, HEAVEN DEFEND ME AGAINST
THE HERESY! I may be a doctor or some new kind of
specialist that will someday receive an appropriate name—
a specialist in the human heart and human behavior. But
not a judge (Lindsey & Borough, 1931, p. 315).

So wrote Judge Ben B. Lindsey, who singlehandedly created a Juvenile
and Family Relations Court in Denver. He thought of his court, which
began functioning almost simultaneously with the Chicago Court, as
an "institution of human relations (misnamed a court)," designed not
to punish people, but to help them. In his court, "the human artist
succeeded the executioner." Not only did Lindsey think of the court
as a strategically located helping agency, but he succeeded in making
his court a place where children voluntarily came for help. He sent
hundreds of juveniles to reform school and prison without escort and
without the loss of a single prisoner; the rate of commitment to institutions of those on probation was 3 percent; and there is some
suggestion that at least in the early years of the operation of his court
there was a positive reduction in delinquent acts in the community.
Lindsey was internationally renowned as a founder of the juvenile
court system, and although his clinical contributions have been lost,

185

his many contributions in law are immortalized in statute and precedent. Lindsey was a powerful clinical therapist because he was also a powerful social therapist. His power to reach individuals came about because his court was firmly embedded in his community. He understood his community and the culture of the children with whom he worked and he used both as helping tools. A shrewd, able politician of unimpeachable integrity, he enhanced his role as judge by working selflessly and fearlessly for political and social reforms to benefit the people of his city.

In this chapter we describe Lindsey's methods, for although the man himself was unique, there are many aspects of his approach which exemplify important social and clinical principles. Lindsey had an informal manner, he modified many court procedures, and he placed many children on probation.[1] His desire to help was coupled with a subtle understanding of the children with whom he worked, and with intensive and personal follow-up of the work he started in the court.

Lindsey's Denver court cannot be divorced from either the man or the city of his day, so it behooves us to examine both in order to appreciate fully Lindsey's approach.

Denver at the turn of the century

Denver came into being during the Pike's Peak gold rush in 1859; for forty years thereafter it was wild and woolly, experiencing fire and flood, boom and bust, and mushroom-like growth. When gold was discovered in the area in 1859, prospectors used Denver as headquarters to purchase supplies, to conduct other business, and for recreation. After the Civil War the railroads came west, and as early as 1872 Denver was a center for four companies. Lindsey's father came

[1] Unfortunately many juvenile courts, even those established in the early years, adopted the informality of procedure but not the substance of Lindsey's "human artistry." Recently the Supreme Court said about the Juvenile Court that it does not treat but violates the constitutional rights of individuals who appear before it and it should be strongly modified. Polier's (1964) survey of the operation and effectiveness of New York's Juvenile Court system provides some indication of why criticism of the Juvenile Court is warranted. Serious criticism was directed at the Juvenile Court concept very early, for very similar reasons (Eliot, 1914).

to Denver to work for one of the railroads. While the population of Denver was only 4,759 in 1870, by 1880, when Lindsey's family arrived, the population had jumped to 34,555. The gold rush had petered out earlier, but in 1880 silver was discovered, and from that point on Denver's growth in population and in industry was spectacular. By 1890, the population was 106,000; by 1900, 133,000, and by 1910, it was 213,000.

Denver was a mining territory (Colorado did not become a state until 1876), peopled by tough pioneers and adventurers, squatters and claim-jumpers eager for riches. A loose but somewhat complex legal system was in operation until the 1890's when the state legislature began to revise it. Outlaws were not uncommon in the area and legally constituted authority was often supplemented by vigilante law. As late as 1878, the Indian agent in the area, an army general, and an army major were killed in a minor Indian uprising. The city catered to the desire for excitement, and bars, dance halls, and gambling were prominent local industries. Even the *Rocky Mountain News,* in an anniversary edition meant to celebrate Denver romantically, characterized the theatres of the time as "somewhat rowdy." They were basically drinking establishments with theatres on the second floor.

The discovery of silver in 1880 made mining and metal refining major industries. Private mints for coinage had been established earlier to solve the problem of transporting gold dust. In addition to mining and related industries, a wholesale trade grew, and railroading became an important source of employment. By 1926, Denver was served by nine roads. After 1880, as the only large city in a 500-mile radius, Denver was established as an industrial and commercial center.

The population growth which accompanied industrialization and urbanization came largely from migrants going west, but there were also a fair number of immigrants. In 1900, when the population of Denver was 133,000, there were about 25,000 foreign-born individuals. Most of them came from England, Ireland, Scotland, Germany, and Sweden. There were only 1,500 or so Russian-born individuals in Denver at that time. There was an insufficient number from other Eastern or Southern European countries to be listed separately, even though Lindsey did speak of sections of Denver called "Little Israel" and "Little Italy." There were only 3,300 Negroes in Denver, for it had never been involved in the slave trade in pre-Civil War days.

The ethnic and national composition of Denver's population is important to note since cultural differences between the majority and minority groups were probably less pronounced here than on the Eastern seaboard. This factor may have helped Lindsay to gain support for his work in the community since there was no American-born majority to complain of "foreigners" who created problems in their city.

The newness of many of the formal institutions of Denver is another factor which may have been important in Lindsey's success in gaining widespread community support. With the growth of industry and population, Denver began to settle down. The Denver Bar Association was formed in 1891, at about the time a series of important reforms were introduced into the judicial system. The state reformatory was established in 1890 and a state industrial school for boys in 1891. The school system was also relatively new, having really begun as a public system in the early 1870's. The absence of long tradition may have made it easy for the schools to adopt modern practices. Denver's public schools in the 1880's and 1890's already included health education, home economics, industrial arts, music, art, and modern languages in the curriculum, subjects which schools in the rest of the nation did not adopt until many years later. A school law designed in part to strengthen the school's hand in dealing with truants and disciplinary problems was passed in April, 1899. It was this law which Lindsey used in establishing his court.

The city of Denver did not receive its municipal charter until 1902, shortly after Lindsey began the Juvenile Court. In Denver, the Juvenile Court was not only part of the general reform movement of the period; it seems also to have been part of the establishment of legitimate forms of institutionalized social controls in a city that was ready to stabilize.

Lindsey the man

Throughout his forty-year career, Lindsey lived the "Dangerous Life," by which he meant that he exposed himself to great professional and personal risk to stand for what he believed was right. At various times in his career, in a variety of combinations, he took on the trusts, corrupt politicians, the Republican party, the Democratic party, the

Bar Association, the Colorado Supreme Court, the sheriffs and police, the penal system, social workers (he called them "scientific robots"), civic groups, patriotic societies, the Ku Klux Klan, and the church. He braved personal insult and threats to his life and livelihood and fought legislative investigations, smears, and frameups until his political enemies succeeded in disbarring him from practicing law while on the bench.[2]

In the 1920's he achieved notoriety for his advocacy of companionate marriage, a set of concepts about marital and sexual relationships that derived from his experience in the Juvenile and Family Relations Court. Fervent opposition was stirred by his proposals for liberalized and realistic divorce laws, for sex education in the schools for children and adults, and for the repeal of anti-birth control laws (Lindsey & Evans, 1925). He was accused by the clergy, physicians, and others of promoting "trial marriage," a concept which he actually opposed.

Never one to back away from a battle, Lindsey used every public relations weapon he could to express his views and to promote his causes. Because of his ingenuity in gaining publicity, he developed a reputation as a grandstander. Even today, some professionals will assert that his achievements were more in the realm of publicity than in the realm of actuality. However, such an assertion overlooks the many reforms in law he actually accomplished, and as we shall see, is false with respect to his clinical accomplishments while on the court.

Lindsey was born in Tennessee in 1869. His father, a dashing Confederate captain and an intellectual, was manager for Western Union in his town. His mother was a true southern belle, noted for her Irish beauty and wit. She was born and raised on a typical plantation, in a great manor house which both before and after the Civil War was the gathering place for young officers of the Confederacy and their ladies.

---

[2] He was disbarred in 1929 because he had acted as a mediator in the case of a disputed will in New York City. The case was not in his jurisdiction in Colorado and had nothing to do with his court. From the autobiographical account, it appears that political enemies got him on a very shaky technicality. Subsequent to his disbarment in Colorado he practiced law in California, and later was elected to a six-year term as Judge of the Los Angeles Superior Court. The Supreme Court of Colorado offered to reinstate him if he apologized for statements he made about the court in one of his books. Characteristically, Lindsey refused, saying the court's offer itself vindicated him. He was restored to the Colorado bar several years later (Lindsey & Borough, 1931; *New York Times*, March 27, 1943).

Married after the Civil War, his mother and father lived on the plantation. Lindsey's grandfather, who owned the plantation, was a powerful, bluff man of impeccable standards. As foreman of the grand jury in his area, he explosively denounced what was crooked or underhanded in public life. He considered himself a free thinker and described his own ancestors as "free booters." Apparently the Civil War did not drastically affect the family's style of life. Lindsey and his brother were raised on the plantation. They had a colored "Mammy," played and lived with Negro children, and enjoyed the farm, the animals, and the countryside. The family was apparently well-to-do, even in the Reconstruction period, for Lindsey states that his mother lived an easy life with many servants.

His father must have been a restless man for he converted to Catholicism after Lindsey was old enough to recall his father's participation in the Episcopalian Church. His mother also converted, and Lindsey was sent to a parochial school. The family's Catholicism was sufficient cause for the family to be near ostracized in a Southern Baptist community. The community's reaction to the family may have been a factor in the decision to go West. When the West opened up and the railroads needed telegraphers, his father accepted a position in Denver and relocated the family in 1879, when Lindsey was ten.

For a while the move went well for the Lindseys. Lindsey and his brother were sent to the Notre Dame prep school where he learned to debate and where he experienced a variety of religious crises. He studied the lives of the saints and was considered a promising candidate for the priesthood. However, while the boys were at school, their father lost his job, became ill, and fell into debt. Lindsey returned to Tennessee to the plantation, and continued in a Baptist school, where he persisted in both his Catholicism and his debating. A few years later, he rejoined his family in Denver, but his father's health was poor and Lindsey went to work to help support the family. He was not even able to attend the Denver High School.

Lindsey made up his mind to study the law and at 17 he finally secured a position as an office boy with a lawyer. In addition to working and trying to study law, Lindsey supplemented his income by selling newspapers and by doing janitorial work at night. Shortly afterwards, his father died penniless, one day after his insurance lapsed because he had neglected to pay the last premium. At one point, Lindsey was so despondent that he attempted suicide and was saved only because the cartridge in his revolver failed to explode.

The failure of his suicide attempt enabled Lindsey to face life with renewed vigor and he returned to his work and to the study of law. By 1894, he was admitted to the bar. As a young lawyer he was appointed attorney to defend two small boys who had been arrested as burglars and who were in a cell with adult criminals. His defense of the boys included a public indictment against the state's treatment of these children and won him some popular attention.

Later he entered into a law partnership with a man who became a state senator, and in the course of the partnership, he participated in Denver politics. Lindsey proved to be an excellent party worker, although he fast became disillusioned with the chicanery he encountered. He advanced in Democratic party councils to the point where he was able to command consideration for the district attorney's office. He did not receive the nomination for district attorney, but instead he was appointed county judge to fulfill the remaining months of the term of a man who with his help had won election to the State Supreme Court. In January, 1901, Lindsey took office as judge and terminated his law practice.

the beginning of the Juvenile Court

While hearing a civil case, the assistant district attorney asked him if he would interrupt the proceedings for a few minutes to dispose of a larceny case. A boy had been caught stealing coal from the railroad, and he had no defense. Under the law, Lindsey was obliged to sentence the boy to the State Reform School. As he did, the boy's mother, who was in court, began to scream. Lindsey was so touched by the woman's anguish that he arranged for a suspended sentence. That night, Lindsey went to the boy's home, and there discovered the utter poverty of the family. The father was ill of lead poisoning, an occupational disease he had acquired in his work in the smelters. The family was cold.

With the injustice of the case still in mind, Lindsey heard another case of three boys charged with burglary of some pigeons from a man whom Lindsey knew from his own youth to be a grouch and a target of boyish mischief. The boys had been brought into court on criminal charges. Investigating, he learned that officers of the court were paid fees for each conviction. When they wished to replenish the fees account, they simply rounded up children in the city and brought them into court on criminal charges. His indignation aroused, he began looking into the problem of the treatment of children by the police and the courts and the more he found, the more concerned he became. He visited the jails, compiled statistics about treatment of children by the courts and the prisons, and he searched the statute books for laws which might be useful in helping children in trouble. He did find a section of the Colorado School Law of 1899 under which it was possible to treat children in trouble as "juvenile disorderly persons" and not as criminals. The district attorney agreed to file all complaints against children under this law in Lindsey's court. That action was the beginning of the Juvenile Court in Denver.

In part, Lindsey decided on a course of probation because of the abominable conditions existing in the prisons and reform schools. He worked very hard and very effectively to get school boards to appoint truant officers whom he could also use as court probation officers. His use of the school law to justify the court probably helped involve the schools in the court's work. In the next few months Lindsey spoke to countless groups of schoolteachers, women's clubs, church groups, charitable societies, and community organizations to bring to public consciousness the problem of the children. He attracted a great deal of attention to his court, and his clear desire to help won him the cooperation of parents whose children got into trouble. Lindsey wanted to use popular support to gain leverage for a variety of reform laws he was drafting.

Lindsey as a social reformer

Earlier he had made political enemies when he refused to participate in shady propositions involving his court and when he refused to cooperate in making patronage appointments to the court's staff. A few months before the 1901 election he heard the case of a saloon keeper who was selling liquor illegally and who was involved with prostitution. The man paid protection to the political powers and fully expected to be acquitted. Lindsey convicted him. While he brought himself to the favorable attention of the reformers who were trying to help Denver settle down, he marked himself with politicians as a man who would not play the game. The machine politicians could not prevent Lindsey's renomination in 1901, but they attempted to elect his Republican opponent. Lindsey, however, had built a broad base of popular support, and the people of Denver rallied to save "the kid's court." He ran 2,000 votes ahead of his ticket, and thus found himself in a position of political power and independence.

From his vantage point in the County Court, Lindsey began to press for a variety of reforms. He wanted a law to prevent politicians from exploiting the estates of widows and orphans and another to forbid the collection of fees for prosecuting children. He eventually obtained a contributory juvenile delinquency law to prosecute neglectful parents and other adults who seduced children into trouble; a Juvenile Court law with probation officers who had police powers; and a detention school to hold children. He pressed for improved child labor laws and for the enforcement of the compulsory school attendance law. He worked for public baths, public playgrounds, and for trade schools.

In his fight for these laws, Lindsey went into the gambling dens, the saloons, the houses of prostitution, and the factories and he saw for himself what was happening. He publicized what he saw in speeches, newspaper interviews, and occasional columns. When he found out the district attorney's office would not prosecute the gamblers, Lindsey invited the Board of Police Commissioners to his court. He informed the newspapers, and then publicly accused members of the board of knowingly permitting the ruination of children, of being personally responsible for the appalling immorality which came before his court. The newspapers spread the story, the ministers took up the cry, and as the worst of the dives shut their doors, Lindsey went to the legislature to obtain his contributory delinquency laws and police power for the probation officers of his court.

Lindsey wanted to obtain a detention home-school because he found conditions in the jails were almost as abominable as they were in the dives. Children learned to become criminals from adult criminals, they were subject to homosexual assaults, engaged in homosexual activity among themselves, and managed somehow to contact the women and girls who were also confined in the jail. When released, Lindsey felt the children went back to their schools and then introduced others to practices they had learned. Lindsey also found that children were frequently abused physically by the police. As a result of their confinement, many came to look upon the law as a hated enemy.

His attempts to obtain prison reform laws were sabotaged in the legislature not by open opposition, but by legislative skulduggery, so Lindsey again went to the public. He arranged for an interview with a friendly reporter who wrote a front page story detailing the variety of horrors encountered in the jails. When the police commissioners denied Lindsey's charges, he demanded an open investigation, and set a meeting in his court to which he invited the governor, the mayor, fifteen prominent ministers, the police board and members of the city council.

Lindsey attempted to subpoena witnesses for this hearing but the subpoenas were never officially served. Lindsey then turned to Mickey, "the worst kid in town." Mickey, who was a leader among the children, was working with Lindsey to organize a newsboys' association under the court's supervision. When told of Lindsey's dilemma, Mickey rounded up twenty boys who had been in jail, herded them into the court for the hearing, and at Lindsey's invitation acted as an assistant by selecting the order of witnesses to be heard by the investigating body.[3] The boys detailed their experience in the jails and with the police. As a result of the investigation, Lindsey gained further support from the ministers and from the governor of the state. With the subsequent publicity, he was able to get the state legislature to pass his Juvenile Court bills.

His fight for public playgrounds took somewhat the same course. Two years of public agitation (newspaper articles, speeches, appeals to the city council, formation of a juvenile improvement association) were necessary to win playgrounds. The case for public baths was won when Lindsey encouraged his boys to swim in bathing suits in the bronze-cherubed fountains in front of the courthouse. When the police chased them, the boys ran dripping into the courtroom for Lindsey's protection. His tactics persuaded the city council to see that if the city could afford decorative fountains, it could also afford free public baths for those who needed them.

Lindsey's court uncovered a grafting scandal which reached to the Board of County Commissioners and which involved a number of respectable businessmen. Although there was considerable pressure on him to back away, he pursued the issue and obtained convictions. About

---

[3] Lindsey frequently used children as unofficial agents of the court and he frequently used their gangs to do the work of delinquency prevention. In subsequent sections, we shall give some further description of Lindsey's relationship to the children's gangs of Denver. Let it suffice here to quote Lincoln Steffens, who said Lindsey was "the leader of every kid's gang in Denver" (Steffens, 1909).

the same time, Lindsey investigated conditions in the cotton mills which opened just outside of Denver. He visited the factories and the homes and he talked with the children. When he became convinced children were being illegally exploited, he saw to it the company was prosecuted. Not only did he prosecute the superintendent of the mill but he also insisted on fining the owner. The mill moved out of town and Lindsey incurred the wrath of a portion of the business community.

In the election of 1904, Lindsey had the support of the Women's Clubs of Denver, the newsboys, who openly campaigned on Denver's streets for "our little Ben," and the ministers. He managed to gain the nominations of both major parties, against the opposition of political bosses. Although he won, technical legal considerations forced him into another election which proved to be extraordinarily dirty. Lindsey came out on top, and subsequently he got into a variety of battles with the utilities, the railroads, the water company, and other "interests." Lindsey carried some of the prosecutions of the "interests" through his own court, and in his book, *The Beast* (Lindsey & O'Higgins, 1910), he exposed other aspects of corporation corruption.

As part of his battle, Lindsey worked to reform the election laws, "to restore the tools of democracy to the people," and in retaliation, the political bosses tried to pass bills which would have undercut his position as county judge. Again, rallying the support of newspapers, the newsboys, and the Women's Clubs, Lindsey beat down the attempt to get him and managed to win some election reforms. His battles against the corporations kept him constantly in the public eye. In 1908, when the political bosses succeeded in keeping the nomination of both parties from him, he ran as an independent, gaining widespread support because of his efforts at political reform and his work on the Juvenile Court. He was elected with a vote almost as great as the total received by his opponents on the Democratic and Republican tickets.

Lindsey continued to win election or appointment regularly until he finally was deprived of his position on the court by the State Supreme Court which threw out the results of the 1924 election on technical grounds. In 1924 the KKK was riding high in Denver and Lindsey was a prime target. He was later disbarred by that same court, so that he never again could serve the Juvenile and Family Relations Court in Denver. By 1927, his ideas on companionate marriage had made him notorious and lost him much of the support he had previously commanded among the clergy.

Through these years Lindsey became a world-renowned figure, speaking and writing about the Juvenile Court. There were numerous magazine articles by him and about him in both professional and popular periodicals. The *Ladies' Home Journal, McCall's, Everyman's, Outlook,* and the *Literary Digest* regularly carried features about Lindsey. He was unquestionably known and widely respected throughout the country, although it is interesting that one writer stated he was better thought of in the East than in the West.

It is important to record Lindsey's political history in order to fully understand the operation of his Juvenile Court. His effectiveness as a Juvenile Court judge was due to more than his informal approach and his reliance on probation. These techniques were adopted by other, less successful, courts. His effectiveness came about because he was committed to helping the people battle against forces which were hurting them. In his political role, Lindsey gave the disenfranchised a stake in government and he made the facilities of his court available to children so that they could obtain redress for their grievances. In electing Lindsey, people of Denver were truly electing their own representative. Clearly, the attitude that was held toward Lindsey as a political agent extended to Lindsey as a helping agent. If he was on the side of the people in his political attacks on their oppressors, then in his work in the court, he could not have been perceived solely as an agent of society bent on controlling and punishing the deviate. In his work on the court, Lindsey was viewed as a person who wanted to help, and in his hands the court became a helping agency. His manner and methods on the court and his political and reform activities supplemented and validated each other.

Not only was Lindsey's court embedded in the community by his political activities; it was also embedded in the community by his helping methods. Lindsey related the work of the court to the work of the schools and he used his knowledge of individuals and of groups to foster the work of the court. Children became agents of the court. This action provided a form of delinquency control in the very agency which had formerly served only to punish and to exclude from society.

the effectiveness of his work

How does one evaluate the effectiveness of an institution? Is its humaneness as important as the concrete results it achieves? Can one evaluate the court in terms of dollars and cents, as Lindsey does in one article? Is the purpose of the court to prevent the development of adult criminal careers? It is difficult to say, obviously. And even if one could say the purpose was to prevent delinquency or adult criminal careers, it is not clear the relevant variables are understood sufficiently to make a fair evaluation possible.

In Lindsey's day, before the Juvenile Court, children were thrown in jail. The effectiveness of the probation system could be tested by seeing how many children who were placed on probation were eventually committed to the State Industrial School. Scattered figures are available for Lindsey's court and for several other juvenile courts of the day, but the comparability of the figures is very poor. They are taken to different base lines and cover varying time periods. Frequently there is no rhyme or reason in reporting data for five months, fifteen months, or two years. It is as if the various courts haphazardly selected figures for the sake of a public report. The criteria used in deciding when a child had committed a sufficiently serious breach of probation to warrant incarceration were never explicit. The attitude of the judge is tremendously important, as Polier (1964) has shown for modern juvenile courts. An extreme example is found in the St. Louis judge who seemed to have an unreasoning prejudice against an early probation law governing treatment of juveniles. In a year and a half, this judge placed only one boy on probation (International Prison Commission, 1904, p. 163). The availability of facilities for incarceration is still another issue (Polier, 1964).

Despite all of these limitations, which should be kept clearly in mind, we will report some of the figures from the early juvenile courts to give some basis for comparison, however poor, with the present time. Clearly, if one is to consider seriously the model presented by Lindsey's court and other courts, one must ask what they actually accomplished by their approach. Other values will become clear in our further discussion below.

Let us first offer some figures from various juvenile courts and then concentrate on the figures Lindsey provides for the first three years of his court. Records from the Chicago Juvenile Court for 1903 show that 1,301 cases were adjudicated over a nine-month period. Of these, 715 were placed on probation, but 505, nearly all repeated offenders, were sent to the John Worthy School, an institution with a reputation for strict discipline. There is no way of estimating the percent of probation violations within any one year from these data, but one can safely estimate it is probably no lower than 33 percent. For the year 1903 in New York, 13.1 percent of children on probation were subsequently committed for violation of probation. In the Philadelphia Court, for 17 months, from June, 1901, to November, 1902, no more than 27 cases of 1,008 placed on probation returned to appear before the court more than once. In that same court, from October, 1903, to January, 1904, of 367 under probation, only 22 returned to the court two or more times. (Why these odd periods are presented is unclear, and the data are presented in such fashion that it is very difficult to evaluate their exact significance.) In St. Louis, in a five-month period, less than 8 percent were returned to the court for sentencing after they had been placed on probation (International Prison Commission, 1904). As late as 1925, Hoffman claimed there were only six Cincinnati boys, of a population of 1,200, in the State Reform School (Hoffman, 1925, p. 259). None of these figures give any indication of repeated offenses committed by the children on probation, nor do they tell us anything about the number of children who later became adult criminals. For the sake of rough comparability, we may look at figures summarized by Sutherland and Cressey (1960) for more recent times. They cite delinquency recidivist rates of no lower than 25 percent and as high as 88 percent for a five-year period. Other sources (Juvenile Court Statistics, 1963) suggest that about 20 percent of all children on probation violate the conditions of probation and are returned to the Juvenile Court. In all, then, in comparison, there is some suggestion the early courts did have some effectiveness with their children.[4]

Lindsey presents data which are somewhat more clear-cut in a report authored by him and his probation staff entitled *The Problem of the Children and How the State of Colorado Cares for Them* (Lindsey,

---

[4] It is instructive to note that Chicago, the court with the poorest record, had civil service probation workers who complained even then they did not have adequate time to supervise their probationers. Philadelphia had a decentralized, privately supported probation officer system, with the workers, all women, selected by the New Century Club, a women's group. The Indianapolis Court made extensive use of volunteers for probation work as did Hoffman in Cincinnati. Hoffman says, "It has been tacitly, if not expressly, determined by the social agencies of Cincinnati, the public schools and all the civic organizations that no child manifesting symptoms of conduct disorders shall enter a criminal career" (Hoffman, 1925, p. 259). The volunteer system and the Big Brother movement were used extensively by the early courts (Coulter, 1913). Problems in the use of volunteers are discussed by Rogers of the Indianapolis Court (International Prison Commission, 1904) and by Eliot (1914).

1904). The report was prepared to answer requests for information about the Juvenile Court, and in part it was designed to be distributed at the Denver Juvenile Court Exhibit at the St. Louis World's Fair of 1904. The bulk of the document also appears as part of the report of the International Prison Commission (1904) to the Congress of the United States. The fact that the report was used for such varied purposes is important in evaluating its significance. We have been unable to locate any independent statistical survey of the effectiveness of Lindsey's court and it is necessary to rely on the figures he offers. We shall cite these as background for a description of the operation of his court, and not as definitive evidence of the effectiveness of that court.

In the first two years of the operation of the Denver Juvenile Court, 715 children were brought before the court for delinquency. Of this total, 554 were placed on probation while 40 were forthwith committed to the State Industrial School. (The disposition of the remainder of the cases is not clear. Some were dismissed, while others were remanded to their parents' custody.) Of the 554 on probation, only 31 committed offenses of such a character as to require commitment to the State Industrial School. For the two-year period, 1902–1903 (the data overlap with the material reported above), 719 cases were heard. The vast bulk of these were placed on probation and in the two-year period, only 23 children committed further offenses serious enough to warrant commitment. These 23 constituted 3.2 percent of the cases placed on probation. Lindsey does not tell us how many children appeared before the courts more than once, and, of course, there is no way of measuring hidden delinquency, but Lindsey asserts that ". . . 95 percent have not committed a second offense, after a period of one to three years . . . " (Lindsey, 1904, p. 35).[5] He goes on to say that over 50 percent of all the boys discharged from the courts before the existence of the Juvenile Court did commit further offenses within comparable periods of time. A political pamphlet (1913) quotes the warden of the state penitentiary who said that in 13 years of the court's existence, only three who were in the state penitentiary had ever been in Juvenile Court.

In that same 1904 report, there is some evidence that Lindsey's court had a positive effect in reducing delinquency in the community. The matron of the police department writes in 1904: "We do not have half as many boys placed under our care by the police as we did two

[5] In later years he reduced this estimate to 80 to 90 percent.

years ago, and I attribute the fact to the manner in which the Juvenile Court is conducted" (p. 185). Endorsements of his work by several police chiefs are also found in later political pamphlets collated by the Denver Public Library.

The Chief Officer of the Special Secret Service of the Union Pacific Railroad Company wrote in the 1904 report:

> The railroad companies have for years been subject to depredations of boys, who have committed all sorts of depredations against the property of the company from breaking into cars and robbing them of their contents and the stealing of brass attachments off the cars. . . . our trouble with this class of offenders has been largely and almost entirely done away with. *In fact, our* losses from this class of thieves have been reduced *at least ninety percent,* and the boys who formerly were ringleaders and really caused these depredations are now seldom seen around our tracks or property of the company, and on each of the reporting days in your Court I can point out the boys who have caused all this trouble (p. 185).[6]

A similar statement is made by the Special Services Officer of the Colorado and Southern Railroad (p. 189). In 1913, a political pamphlet cites a letter from a railroad officer who stated that in a three-year follow-up of 97 boys he had referred to the court because of delinquencies against the railroad, he had repeated complaints against only two boys.

The Denver Department Stores Detective said:

> It gives me unqualified satisfaction to inform you that none of your wards have left their reservation for a long time, and that the part of the city known as department stores, which until last year were their supposed privileged grounds, have not even seen a hunting party. We can now turn out our toy play sheep, tin soldiers and woolly dogs, bears, wild cats, deer, etc., without fear of loss or molestation. We even dare to leave children's marbles, spring guns,

[6] The railroad officers apparently were invited to appear in court on reporting days, an event to be described fully below.

locomotives, trains of cars and candy carelessly about, and none, so far, have been missing. This line of stock, as you may imagine, has always had a peculiar fascination for some of our youngsters and I cannot quite understand the influence you must have brought to bear on them that such magnificent results have been attained (p. 186).

Similar statements of unqualified support are presented in the 1904 report by a number of school superintendents, principals, and teachers, and numerous editorials are quoted from the Denver papers of 1904. The editorials of that day might be compared with the periodic outcries against the juvenile courts in almost all of today's newspapers.

Lindsey's probation system

In subsequent pages, we shall try to present Lindsey's system. Many of the quotations we will use to illustrate his methods read like movie scripts. They are not accurate transcripts. O'Higgins, one of Lindsey's collaborators (Lindsey and O'Higgins, 1910), was a professional writer. He was on the staff of *Everybody's Magazine* and was sent by the magazine to prepare a series of articles with Lindsey. The material in the book was reworked from Lindsey's dictated notes. Borough, another of his coauthors (Lindsey & Borough, 1931), was a newspaper editor who also worked from notes dictated to him by Lindsey. Borough (personal communication) had the advantage of seeing Lindsey at work in the Los Angeles Court. He took shorthand notes of Lindsey's interview with a young tough. There are also first-hand journalistic accounts by men as distinguished as Lincoln Steffens (1909), Franklin P. Adams (*Literary Digest*, 1915). and William McLeod Raine (1907) of Lindsey's approach in his court, and these accounts differ very little qualitatively from Lindsey's autobiographical accounts of his techniques. Lindsey the man and his basic approach come through with such clarity that it seems worthwhile quoting extensively from these various accounts.

When a child was brought to the court, he was classified as either a schoolchild or a working child. If in school, information about his school, his teacher, his neighborhood, his home, and his parents would be obtained. If a child was working, the court determined the nature of his employment, and if he was unemployed, the court would make an effort to assist him in obtaining employment.

When he appeared in court, a child was informed in firm but kindly terms of his obligation to obey the law and to respect authority in the home and in school. The child was told that he "must overcome evil with good and make up for his delinquency by being just as decent and good as he can in the home, the neighborhood and the school." A child placed on probation was given the implicit trust and confidence of the court and an effort was made to have him feel that his failure would "let the judge down."

On the other hand, the child was asked to provide evidence of being worthy of this trust and confidence.

> We impress him with the idea that we have no doubt whatever that he will keep his word, that he will respect his honor and the confidence we have put in him, and that no one will question his doing it, and that we have a record of that fact, we ask the boy himself voluntarily to get a report from his teacher every other Friday preceding the session of the Juvenile Court every other Saturday. This report is made upon a printed card, and details conduct in school and school attendance. It is graded: excellent, good, fair and poor. It is soon understood that "good" is satisfactory, "fair" is passable, "excellent" is particularly pleasing to us, and "poor" is very displeasing. Any boy that brings a poor report at the morning session is made to understand that it is "not square" (Lindsey, 1904, p. 72).

The actual operation of the Saturday morning sessions was vastly different in tone from Lindsey's description above. Lindsey discussed his report system with Lincoln Steffens.

> "What I was after," the Judge explained, "was something for which I could praise the boy in open court. Believing in approbation as an incentive, I had to have their reports for the boy to show me in order that I might have a basis for encouraging comment, or, if the reports were not up to

the mark, for sympathy. It didn't matter to me very much what the reports were about. . . . But you can see that these fortnightly reports were an excuse for keeping up my friendly relationship with the boy, holding his loyalty, and maintaining our common interest in the *game of correction* [italics added] he and I were playing together" (Steffens, 1909, p. 132).

the Saturday morning report session

Fortunately, Steffens provides a detailed description of the Saturday morning report sessions. It will be seen that Lindsey practiced a form of group therapy in his court, in which his charges were restored to a state of grace in the community.

> The boys assemble early, two or three hundred of them, of all ages and all sorts, "small kids" and "big fellers"; well dressed "lads" and ragged "little shavers"; burglars who have entered a store, and burglars who have "robbed back" pigeons; thieves who have stolen bicycles, and thieves who have "swiped" papers; "toughs" who have "sassed" a cop or stoned a conductor, and boys who have talked bad language to little girls, or who "hate their father," or who have been backward at school and played hookey because the teacher doesn't like them. It isn't generally known, and the Judge rarely tells just what a boy has done; the deed doesn't matter, you know, only the boy, and all boys look pretty much alike to the Judge and to the boys. So they all come together there, except that the boys who work, and newsboys, when there's an extra out, are excused to come at another time. But nine o'clock Saturday morning finds most of the "fellers" in their seats, looking as clean as possible, and happy.
>
> The Judge comes in and, passing the bench, which looms up empty and useless behind him, he takes his place, leaning against the clerk's table or sitting on a camp chair.

"Boys," he begins, "last time I told you about Kid Dawson and some other boys who used to be with us here and 'who made good'. Today I've got a letter from the Kid. He's in Oregon, and he's doing well. I'll read you what he says about himself and his new job."

And he reads the letter which is full of details roughly set in a general feeling of encouragement and self-confidence.

"Fine, isn't it!" the Judge says. "Kid Dawson had a mighty hard time with himself for awhile, but you can see he's got his hand on the throttle now. Well let's see. The last time I talked about snitching, didn't I? Today, I'm going to talk about 'ditching.'" And he is off on the address, with which he opens court. His topics are always interesting to boys, for he handles his subjects boy-fashion. "Snitching", the favorite theme, deals with the difference between "snitching" which is telling on another boy to hurt him; and "snitching on the square," which is intended to help the other fellow. "Ditching" is another popular subject. "To ditch" a thing is to throw it away; and the Judge, starting off with stories of boys who have ditched their commitment papers,[7] proceeds to tell about others who, "like Kid Dawson out there in Oregon" have "ditched" their bad habits and "get strong." I heard him on Arbor Day speak on trees; how they grow some straight, some crooked. There's always a moral in these talks, but the judge makes it plain and blunt; he doesn't "rub it in."

After the address, which is never long, the boys are called up by schools. Each boy is greeted by himself, but the judge uses only his given or nickname. "The boys from the Arapahoe Street School," he calls, and as the group come forward, the Judge reaches out and seizing one by the shoulder, pulls him up to him saying: "Skinny, you've been doing fine lately; had a crackerjack report every time."[8]

---

[7] Lindsey sent boys to the State Industrial School without escort. His approach is described below.

[8] In a typical month, less than 10 percent of the reports were poor while about 7 percent were excellent (Lindsey, 1904). Probation workers today will often avoid contacts with the school because they fear prejudicing teachers against the child who has become involved with the court. Lindsey, on the other hand, consulted

He opens the report. "And you have. That's great. Shake, Skin. You're all right, you are." Skinny shines.

Pointing at another, he says: "And you, Mumps, you got only 'fair' last time. What you got this time? You promised me 'excellent', and I know you've made good." He tears open the envelope. "Sure," he says. "You've done it. Bully for you." Turning to the room, he tells "the fellers" how Mumps began playing hookey, and was so weak he simply thought he couldn't stay in school. "He blamed the teacher; said she was down on him. She wasn't at all. He was just weak, Mumps was; had no backbone at all. But look at him now. He's bracing right up. You watch Mumps. He's the 'stuff' Mumps is. Aren't you Mumps? Teacher likes you now all right, doesn't she? Yes. And she tells me she does. Go on now and keep it up, Mumps. I believe in you."

"Why, Eddie," the Judge says, as another boy came up crying. "What are you crying for? Haven't you made good?"

"No, sir," Eddie says, weeping the harder.

"Well, I told you I thought you'd better go to Golden. You don't want to go, eh? Get another job, you say? But you can't keep it, Eddie. You know you can't. Give you another chance? What's the use, Eddie? You'll lose it. The best thing for you, Eddie, is Golden. They'll help you up there, make you stick to things, just make you; and so you'll get strong."

Eddie swims in tears, and it seemed to me I'd have to give that boy "another chance", but the Judge who is called "easy," was not moved at all.[9] His mind was on the good of that boy; not on his own feelings, nor yet on the boy's. "You see," said he to me, "he is hysterical, ab-

---

teachers and principals concerning the disposition of their children. There was another form of follow-up as well. Teachers knew which of their boys were on probation. If a boy was absent, the teacher would call the probation officer who went out to investigate his absence immediately (Vollmer, 1906).

[9] The Judge had a reputation among the boys for being able to ferret out the truth. He would not accept lies, and he seemed to know instinctively when a boy was not leveling with him. From the point of view of the boys, he was fair, firm, and anything but gullible or soft. Lindsey once said, "Children don't rebel at authority, only ignorant authority" (Steffens, 1909, p. 156).

normal. The discipline of Golden is just what he needs."
And he turned to the room full of boys.

"Boys," he said, "I'm going to send Eddie up to
Golden. He hasn't done wrong; not a thing. But he's weak.
He and I have tried again and again to win out down here
in the city, and he wants another trial. But I think a year
or so at Golden will brace Eddie right up, and make him
a strong manly fellow. He's not going up there to be
punished. That isn't what Eddie needs and that isn't what
Golden is for. Is it, fellers?"[10]

"No, sir," the room shouted.

"It would be unjust to punish Eddie, but Eddie understands that. Don't you, Eddie?"

"Yes sir, but" (blubbering), "Judge, I think if I only
had one more show I could do all right."

"Eddie, you're wrong about that. I'm sure I'm right.
I'm sure that after a year or two you'll be glad I sent you
to the school. And I'll be up there in a few days to see you,
Eddie, myself. What's more, I know some boys up there—
friends of mine, that'll help you Eddie; be friends to you.
They won't like a kid that cries, but I'll tell them you need
friends to strengthen you, and they'll stay with you."[11]

All forenoon this goes on, the boys coming up in
groups to be treated each one by himself. He is known to
the Court, well known, and the Judge, his personal friend,
and the officers of the court and the spectators, his fellow-
clubmen, all rejoice with him, if he is "making good",
and if he is doing badly, they are sorry. And in that case,
he may be invited to a private talk with the Judge, a talk
mind you, which has no terrors for the boy, only comfort.
They often seek such interviews voluntarily. They sneak
into the Judge's chambers or call at his house to "snitch
up" that they are not doing very well. And the boys who

---

[10] His use of the group is critical. Eddie's being sent away to Golden was not an
arbitrary act by the Judge. It was clear to all that Eddie had been given numerous
chances and had not been able to help himself.

[11] Below, in talking about Lindsey's technique in sending boys to Golden without
escort, it will be seen that Lindsey visited the State Industrial School with some
regularity and that he did follow up as he said he would. His visits probably helped
the institution to maintain its standards.

sit there and see this every two weeks; or hear all about it, they not only have forgotten all their fear of the law; they go to the Court now as to a friend, they and their friends. For Judge Lindsey had not been doing "kid justice to kids" very long before all Boyville knew it. The rumor spread like wildfire. The boys "snitched" on the Judge, "snitched on the square"; they told one another that the County Judge was all right (Steffens, 1909, pp. 132–138).

the commitment to help

The report sessions were only one portion of Lindsey's therapeutic program. Lindsey put himself out personally and publicly for his charges. He worked to bring about reforms which were in their interest and in the interest of their families. He made himself available any time, even to the extent of interrupting an adult trial to take care of the business of a child. He was constantly in the neighborhoods, and he frequently visited the homes of the boys. He took them out for meals, to shows, and brought them to his home. In 1915, Lindsey was fined $500 for contempt of court because he refused to reveal information a boy had given him in confidence. The boy was involved in a sensational murder trial, and Lindsey refused to reveal what he knew about the case (*Personal Glimpses*, 1915). In every way he could, he showed concern and a willingness to help, and he made real the principle that the court was acting in the youth's interest.

Lindsey used the court and the facilities of the court to help in a number of ways. The annual report of the probation office for 1903 (Lindsey, 1904) lists 3,139 interviews between the Judge and probationers. Moreover, the court administered 1,150 baths during the year, many of these on report day, in the courthouse basement; provided 252 jobs; provided summer employment for 77 boys;[12] assisted 175

---

[12] The boys went to work in the sugarbeet fields under the supervision of a probation officer. Twenty boys were assigned to each group, and the groups met regularly with the Judge and the probation worker to discuss their work. Judge Lindsey worked to help the boys see their labor was important to the whole state. Compare these groups with the work crew program described by Sarason, et al. (1966). An

children in financial need; and supplied 395 items of clothing both new and used to children. The court had an employment service which was used by non-delinquent children (Lindsey & Evans, 1925). In one instance, Lindsey organized a dancing school so that young people would have a place to go for fun.

The court was used to redress grievances the boys had. In one instance, at a newsboy's request, Lindsey wrote out an "injunction" to get a policeman who had been chasing him from his favorite corner to cease and desist. The boy reported the policeman actually made friends with him after the incident. A probation officer helped a child recover a bike which was stolen from him by an adult. In another instance the court intervened to help a youth who complained that his employer had unfairly deducted money from his salary. In still another case, Lindsey supported the leader of a street gang who got into a fight with a saloon keeper who refused to stop selling liquor to gang members. Lindsey had the saloon keeper arrested and jailed for fifteen days.

In many instances, children came to him themselves to seek help. Often the children who sought him out were adolescent girls who had gotten into sexual difficulty. Lindsey arranged for treatment for children with venereal diseases without necessarily informing their parents or anyone else. He helped pregnant girls in various ways, including arranging for discreet confinement and private adoption of their babies. And all of this was done in the strictest confidence. Lindsey did not approve premarital sexual relationships, but he observed that most of the girls who engaged in premarital sexual relations eventually grew up to be good wives and mothers. It was his feeling that more harm was done by public exposure in the court than by the actual sexual experience. There is no way of knowing how many girls Lindsey helped through the years, for he kept no public record of these cases. In fact, when he left office in 1927, he openly burned his files and records to protect the confidence of untold thousands of children and adults who had trusted him. He burned the records because he did not trust the new chief probation officer, an alleged Ku Klux Klan member (Lindsey & Evans, 1925; Lindsey & Boroughs, 1931; New York Times, 1943).

---

undated political pamphlet, probably prepared in 1912, states that one of Lindsey's major achievements was the development of "a system of cooperative work between the school, the neighborhood, the home, the church, the businessman, and the court in the interest of the child offender."

the reduction of fear

It was not only girls who came to him for help. Lindsey made shrewd use of the desire to confess, the desire to maintain a state of grace, and the psychology of the group in his dealings with children. He worked hard to erase the element of fear from his relationship with a child so that the youngster would be willing to tell him the truth, relieve his conscience, and make amends.

As indicated, Lindsey was not soft, and he did not condone wrongdoing. However, he did not judge and had an unwavering acceptance and respect for the humanness of the individual. He did not become indignant or punitive about sexual or aggressive transgressions, nor about stealing or lying. His attempt was to understand, to accept, and to point the way to an adaptation which would leave the individual with a greater sense of self-worth.

The following excerpt comes from Lindsey's book, *The Dangerous Life*. The reader should again be cautioned that although written as a transcript, it is not a verbatim account. However, the dialogue was written by Rube Borough, who had observed the Judge in action from a concealed vantage point in another case, and it very likely captures the flavor of what went on:

> I recall a type of old time policeman trained alone in the ways of violence bringing a small boy into our court. As the officer came in he glared at the little fellow as though he wanted to eat him up. The boy glared back as though he wanted to throw a brick.
>
> First and foremost, it was evident that no love was lost between the two. The approach in both cases was one of hostility. There is such a thing as human artistry and the greatest of all human artistry, perhaps, is the artistry of approach.
>
> "He is a bad kid" the policeman blurted out, "and there are fifteen or twenty more like him down there about those tracks that I haven't been able to catch because of this kid. For every time I come in sight he is on the lookout and when he sees me coming he yells 'Jigger the Bull!' and everybody scoots and I can't ketch 'em."

This last with an air of offended dignity.

"And when I got this kid, I asks him the names of the kids that run away and he says, 'I dunno 'em. I never saw 'em before.' "

And then as he glared at the boy: "The little liar, he knows every one of 'em.' "

Of course there is no artistry in that method of approach. . . .

I have always made it a rule never to call a boy or girl a liar if it can be avoided—and it generally can. And yet, in the present case, I had to retain the boy's respect for the policeman as the representative of the law as best I could.[13]

"Jimmie," I said with such warmth of smile and attitude as I was able to command, "I am sure you don't understand the officer and he perhaps doesn't understand you. If you did I don't think you would have run away from him and I doubt if he would think that you were really a liar.

"Now, I don't think you are a liar but I do think that you are afraid. The best boy may be afraid when he doesn't understand things. Then when he is afraid he may say things that are not what we call true.

"But that isn't because he wants to lie. It's because he's afraid and thus he doesn't know what else to do. Now don't you think that is true in this case?"

And presently our little prisoner half smiles through his tears and becomes as garrulous as he has been dumb under the menacing glances of his captor.

"It's jest like ye said, Jedge. I ain't no liar and I don't mean to do nothing wrong but I'm just plumb scared."

"Oh yes," I tell him, "I knew you would admit that. You thought you were going to get in jail or the reform school, didn't you? Well, you are not going to get in any such place. You are just going to tell me the truth, for I know you are a truthful boy. We are going to help the

---

[13] Lindsey stood firmly with the law, although he encouraged fights against injustice. When he suggested that a boy who was kept in chains run away from a prison because he knew the guards would not shoot him, he was expressing his indignation at the maltreatment of children.

policeman and the neighborhood and everybody."[14]

"Sure," he says, "I'll tell ye how it was Jedge, I live down there by the railroad tracks, I do, where those kids live. And they said there was watermelons in those boxcars but we didn't find no watermelons.

"But one of de kids sez he bets there is sumpin' good in those boxes 'cause it's got sumpin' on 'em about figs and we think it *is* figs.

"So we gets open a box and finds a lot of bottles with sumpin' on 'em about figs and we thinks it is sumpin' good. So we drinks the whole bottle full. . . ."

And then pausing, he blurts out through his tears: "And I thinks we've done suffered enough."

"Well," I said, "I think so, too, for fig syrup is not recommended in bottle doses."

The policeman doesn't see the humor in this episode that spread about my room and brought titters from the few spectators. Instead he proceeds to gloat over the boy's confession as evidence of the truth of his charge that the boy was a liar, instead of just a frightened kid.

"I told you he was a liar, Judge," he exploded as he turned on the tearful youngster. "Now you know you told me you didn't know anything about any of those kids and you didn't even know their names, but now you tell the judge that you knew them all.

"Now you tell the judge their names—I want their names, see!"

And the little prisoner, hesitating, appeals from policeman to the judge, where somehow he thinks he finds sympathy and understanding, not for his sin but for himself. (For we are dealing much more with him, with what he is than what he did and perhaps why he did it.)

I see the tears come to his eyes again, but he is backed now by a certain confidence as he stands there pleading his own case.

"Do yuh tink, Jedge, that it's square for a guy to snitch on a kid?" he asks.

[14] Lindsey's pitch is to the strength in the boy and to his desire to be accepted in the community.

In some other age of Boyville, if you told or tattled on a boy, you "squealed" and a "squealer" was ever outlawed by the gang. But now if you told on a boy, in the slang or venacular of the gang, you "snitched." And that was against the law. Not our law, but theirs. The first commandment of the gang was—and I suspect ever has been and ever will be—"Thou shalt not snitch (tattle)—you will get your face smashed if you do." *The human quality of loyalty was involved here.*

And unless I had sympathy and understanding for their law, how could I expect them to have sympathy and understanding for mine. [Italics added]

But did this particular type of policeman have any respect for the fact that he was dealing with two worlds and the people that inhabited them and the laws that governed them?

And did he understand that unless he had sympathy and understanding for one he could not expect, much less exact, respect for the other?

The child world and its laws were just as real to Jimmie and as much to be observed and respected as our laws; for they were based on the finest of human qualities, loyalty and respect for each other, however much sometimes through lack of maturity they seem to us to be misdirected. If they are misdirected, the least that can be expected of us is wise direction and not hostility. . . . [15]

---

[15] Lindsey's understanding of the subculture with which he was dealing is beautifully expressed here. Lindsey was sometimes criticized for using boys' language in court, or for not correcting boys' language. His appreciation of the need to communicate in appropriate terms is brought out in the following anecdote which he cites approvingly: Lindsey had worked out an arrangement with the leader of a gang of young Italian Catholics to stop vandalizing a Protestant church located in their neighborhood. The gang had chosen the boy to supervise the protection of the church. The young gang leader tried to get the judge to give him the right to beat up any boys who violated the agreement. Lindsey refused to give him the right, and instead encouraged the boy just to tell his gang.

And following my advice he immediately proceeded to tell the gang, with the accompaniment of the most violent swearing, how he would break their damn necks if they didn't cut it out.

The good old deaconess from the church who had watched these

But to return to our little prisoner—

"Of course, I don't think you should snitch on a kid," I said, "I never asked a boy to snitch on another."

My well meaning friend, the policeman, was unable to restrain at least a mild resentment as he noticed the triumphant look in the face of the little prisoner whose plea had won the aproval of the court.

"Then how do you expect me to get them kids," the policeman inquired. "I been two weeks trying to ketch 'em and now you are going to stand by that kid in his refusal to tell me their names."

"Oh, don't worry about that," I responded. "Jimmie will do more than give us their names. He will bring the boys to court. I am perfectly safe in discharging you from the case with the assurance that we will soon dispose of the lawlessness you have a right to complain about. Isn't that so, Jimmie?"

And there came a curious beam of happy assent from his dirty, grimy little face.

"Sure," he said, through a smile and drying tears. "You betcher life I'll help yuh to stop it, Jedge, if yuh jes' tell me what to do."

"Oh that is easy, Jimmie," I explained. "You go down by the tracks and tell that gang that I have asked Officer Blank to lay off the gang, that I want them to come and see me. I know they will cut it out. After school, tomorrow, you bring them here to see me. They will tell on themselves and you won't have to tell on anybody."

"Sure, I will," said Jimmie, "if I can git 'em to come."

"Well you tell them, and, whatever happens, you just report to me."

And with one final effort to restore peace between the

---

proceedings with undisguised satisfaction, now suddenly screamed in protest, "Judge, stop that boy, he is swearing."

The astonished Tony hesitated as he turned to the lady with the explanation, "Why, don't you want me to tell 'em?"

"Oh, yes, but not to swear at them."

"Well," said Tony, "if I didn't, they wouldn't understand me" (Lindsey & Borough, 1931, p. 136).

little prisoner and the irate officer—which eventually was
to succeed—I was to behold Jimmie leaving the court in
triumph, rather as its agent[16] than its prisoner.

But the next day after school when Jimmie appeared in
my chambers he was alone. He was crestfallen, if not discouraged.

"Well Jimmie," I said, "what's the news from the
front?"

But I was not prepared for the humor of the situation.

"It's like this Jedge," he said. "I tolt those kids you
tolt me to come down and tell 'em to come and see you.
Bud dey wouldn't nobody come. One kid said if his mudder
found out he had been in dis trouble, he would get a good
lickin'. 'Nother said if the cop was goin' to ketch him,
he would have to ketch him. And a big guy said I snitched
on him and he was goin' to beat me up when I never
snitched at all."

Noting the seriousness of this last phase of his experience, I hastened to assure him.

"Of course you didn't snitch, Jimmie," I explained.
"The cop said there were about 15 or 20 boys in that
trouble and we thought it was square to tell how many
without telling any names and you said there were only
seven. Now, I'll tell you, Jimmie. I think the trouble is that
they don't understand. You see, *you* came back. Why?

---

[16] This section provides an excellent example of how Lindsey used the concept of
role in his work with the children. The example also shows how he used the boys
to do the work of the court in the community. We have already told how Mickey
rounded up boys to testify at a hearing Lindsey held to show inequities in the
treatment of children. Mickey was also used to organize children into constructive
activities with the court's support. We have also told how Lindsey delegated "police
authority" to a gang leader to help control vandalism against a Protestant church
in a Catholic neighborhood. In still other instances, Lindsey used boys as unofficial
probation officers, and in the case of Eddie above, Lindsey used the boys in the
state school as his assistants in Eddie's therapy. In Lindsey's numerous battles
with corrupt police and politicians, the boys in the neighborhoods were his eyes
and ears. A policeman taking graft, a dive supposedly closed and then reopened,
saloon keepers who sold liquor to minors or who seduced or forced children into
prostitution became known to Lindsey and he used the information constructively.
In their turn the children campaigned for Lindsey during his election fights and
newsboys shouted "extra" whenever Lindsey wrote a column or a letter to the
editor. In any number of ways Lindsey succeeded in reducing distance by making
the people part of the court, thus encouraging a view of the court as an institution
which helps and not only punishes.

Because you understood and you are not afraid. They did not come because they did not understand and they were afraid."

"Yes," he hastened to inject, "and dey said dey didn't believe that yuh tolt me what you tolt me."

"Oh, I see, you perhaps need some evidence that is more substantial than what you say you told them."

"Sure," he shot back, "Dhat's what I needs. Will you write 'em a note?"

"Sure," I answered, "I'll write them a note. What will I say?"

Jimmie edged up on the table while I took his dictation.

"Tell 'em," he said, "dhat no kid has snitched."

Now self-preservation is the first law of nature and I sympathized with his precaution. Why shouldn't I? Hadn't I been a kid once myself *and who has a right to deal with kids who doesn't remember the days of his childhood?* [Italics added][17]

"And tell 'em," Jimmie went on, as he gained more confidence from this response of sympathy, "if dhey will come to court and promise dhey will cut it out and never do it again yuh won't send 'em up this time."

Consciously or unconsciously, he knew they were afraid and fear is the father of lies, the promotor of lack of confidence between parent and child and cold gulfs that follow and the war of the gang with the police and the war of the nations with each other. For the child's case is the case of all humanity and the cause of evil everywhere. So I wrote the note to the unknown gang.

"Dear Boys," it read, "no kid has snitched. If you will come to the court and promise to cut it out and never do it again I won't send you up this time. Signed, Judge of the Juvenile Court."

That was the warrant and Little Jimmie was the sheriff,[18] [italics added] but he didn't know it. . . .

[17] His ability to empathize with his children is shown clearly in this statement. Borough (personal communication) expressed the opinion that a part of Lindsey always remained a child. He felt that was the reason Lindsey could gain such an immediate rapport with most of the children who came before him.

[18] The use of the concept of role is very clear here.

But our little prisoner, *now our assistant* [italics added], departed right proudly with a warrant of his own dictation. . . .

And I was to find that Jimmie's warrant was so much more effective than that which came down to us from the wigs of the law, even though they were Blackstone, Kent and others. . . .

The next day at the time set for the return of my little friend an officer came in to announce that there was a delegation from the fourth ward waiting outside to see me.

Presently there was ushered in little Jimmie with fourteen as typical ragmuffins from down by the railroad tracks as in my slumming days I had ever gazed upon.

Jimmie was proud and smiling even if the balance of the gang showed timidity—though not without hope, for they trusted Jimmie.

"Well," I said, "Jimmie, you didn't snitch on anybody."

I was looking to his world and the protection he needed there.[19] And it did not go without appreciation as the face of the former little prisoner lighted up and there was a swelling of his chest as he gazed upon the expectant gang.

"But," I continued, "since the policeman said there were about 20 kids in this trouble you thought it would be square to tell how many there were in it really. And you said there were only seven. But you didn't tell the names of any. But, Jimmie, you got fourteen here—how do you account for that?"

"Oh," he answered, "there was only seven of us in it but the rest of dhese kids dhey runs wit' us, dhey does. And dhey got interested in that note of yours and dhey wanted to read it and I let 'em and dhey said dhey would like to come, too. And I said I didn't tink you'd care."

And it was very evident that I did not care before that conference was finished. We not only had the seven who were in it, but the seven who were not in it because they had not had a chance to get in it.

---

[19] Lindsey's remarkable understanding of Jimmie's position in his group is brought out beautifully by this comment.

And then we had a snitching bee, which means that everybody tells on himself and not the other fellow. And since everybody agreed to that—for a sense of real justice is very pronounced in childhood— if you don't keep your word to tell on yourself after you promised to, then you give anybody leave to tell if he is asked. And while that seldom becomes necessary, nevertheless, if it ever does, it is snitching on the square, and you don't get your face smashed for that.

Of course, there was not anything that that gang had ever done that they should not have done that I did not know all about before that conference was finished. All of which proved they were not liars but very truthful little citizens.[20]

We had simply laid the spell of fear and whether in court or home when that is lifted the truth emerges triumphant. Moreover and again, I learned that fear is the father of lies.

And of course, they would cut it out, as indeed they did cut it out—as 99 out of 100 such little citizens did and do when thus approached (Lindsey & Borough, 1931, pp. 120–131).

the power of trust

One of Lindsey's most remarkable achievements was his success in sending hundreds of boys and young men to the state industrial school and to prison by themselves, without escort, and without losing a single prisoner.[21] Lindsey began sending boys to reform school by

[20] Lindsey's use of the term "citizen" should be noted. He includes these children as part of the greater society, not only subject to the coercion of the court, but also privileged to enjoy the benefits of the institutions of the greater society. As a citizen, the child is seen as part of the community.

[21] Lindsey's procedure can be compared with contemporary programs of releasing selected individuals arrested for minor offenses without bail. Ninety-five percent of individuals so treated appear in court at the appropriate time. Most people seem to respond to the trust extended to them.

themselves very early in his career. The 1904 report (Lindsey, 1904) indicates that 18 children had been sent to the State Industrial School in their own custody. Lindsey's action had significance both as a reform of police practice[22] and as a therapeutic tactic. It will be recalled that Lindsey believed that an individual was not evil, but merely weak when he committed an offense. He also believed that each individual had a potential for growth and change which could be reached:

> For I had come to believe that down in every soul, notwith-
> standing the effects of bad environment and the defects of
> heredity, there was what I then chose to call the Image of
> God and it was up to me to bring it out. And my way of

[22] At that time, the sheriffs received a fee for each prisoner delivered to the jails. If a sheriff escorted more than one prisoner on a trip, then he received a fee for each body he delivered. When Lindsey began his practice the sheriffs protested, and several grand jury investigations of his work followed. In one of these investigations, it was brought out that Lindsey had never lost a prisoner he had sent alone, while the sheriffs, who took their prisoners to jail in chains, had had a fair number of successful escapes. Lindsey proposed giving the fee to the boys, but it is not clear that he ever did so (Lindsey, 1904; Lindsey & Borough, 1931).
We have been unable to find any record of a grand jury investigation confirming his claim. However, the claim is repeated over and over in political documents without any indication that his political opponents challenged it. A publication of the Denver Christian Citizenship Union (1910) asserts that the Public Utility Corporation, a political enemy, hired a detective who was unsuccessful in finding anyone to challenge his claim. One undated political pamphlet asserts that Lindsey's court was investigated and exonerated six times, but no specifics are offered. An item in the *Rocky Mountain News*, December 23, 1909, carries statements from police and probation officers denying they or the judge ever accompanied any boy to Golden.
Political enemies charged that Lindsey was too soft on offenders, that his methods encouraged boys to be delinquent because they wanted to be part of the Judge's gang, that no one interfered with his delinquents because they knew Lindsey wouldn't act against the boys, that his tactics undermined respect for parental and school authority, but never that boys ran away when on their honor. The same article claimed that teachers and police couldn't really speak out because they feared reprisals from the politically powerful women's clubs which supported Lindsey (Colorado Humane Society, 1910). On the other hand there are newspaper reports of boys going off on their own, correspondence between reformatory wardens and the Denver Commissioner of Safety referring to such cases (Larsen, 1966, personal communication), and old-time residents of Denver also say he sent boys off alone. The figure of five and then six runaways remains constant in documents from 1910 to 1931. While no one can verify the exact figures, there is little doubt that Lindsey sent hundreds of boys to reform school on their honor, and that he lost few, if any, of these.

attempting to bring it out was, through personal contact, to eliminate hate and fear, instill trust, arouse the desire to please in proving there was one to be pleased, appeal to pride, loyalty, honor. (Lindsey & Borough, 1931, p. 188).

In sending youth to the industrial school in their own custody, Lindsey was appealing to this inner strength. If a youth delivered himself, entered the reform school by virtue of his own will, and proved to himself he could overcome the strongest possible temptation, then he had already performed an act which made his time in the reform school a meaningful part of his rehabilitation. In sending a youth to reform school, Lindsey would discuss the reasons with him and help the boy to see that a term in reform school was the only possible course. As indicated this was often done in public, in court, but it was also done in private conferences with the youngsters.

In the following excerpt Lindsey tells about his first case. He gives us a good view of his approach and an equally good view of his indomitable spirit.

I began to formulate in my own mind an entirely new strategy in dealing with delinquent youth. . . .

If we had to send them to places of artificial restraint, even jails and reformatories, why not send them alone, I asked myself. What stronger proof could I offer to the world of the power of those inner restraints, those forces other than violence, in which I had come to believe?

I discussed the idea with some well meaning friends but they immediately vetoed it as dangerous. Nevertheless, I was determined to put it to the test. And because that seemed to be the least difficult (I afterward found this a mistake), I decided to start with the smaller boys who had to be committed to the detention schools, and the then so-called reform schools.

The very first "culprit" upon whom I tried the experiment, I remember, was a little fellow about 12 years of age. The institution to which he was being sent was located almost on the outskirts of the city. I was sure, I told him before he set forth, that he could be trusted to go alone and "on his honor."

He ran away. The circumstances could not be concealed from the officer who had brought the boy to court in the first place, and there was much merriment around police headquarters at my expense.

I remember the officer said to me, after he had recovered from his gloat of satisfaction over the failure of my experiment:

"I'll catch that little devil and I'll see that he gets what's coming to him—if I have to break his damned neck. You bet I will—no matter what it costs him."

It was not hard to understand the officer's attitude. The youth had been considered an eely little rascal and had been the source of much annoyance to the police through a rather serious type of juvenile burglaries.

But I could not approve of the policeman's program. I thought for a moment and, still fighting for the truth there was in the system I had conceived, I said:

"No, you are wrong. Perhaps you will have to catch him this time. But bring him back to *me* and *I'll* teach him how to be trusted no matter what it costs *me*."[23]

When the little rascal was recovered and brought back to my court by the officer, I found he was fired with hate, not for me but for the officer. His attitude toward me, at first, was one of sham and pretense.

I was learning from the boy—again and again in those days I found that the boys unconsciously taught me more than I could teach them and I often wondered why the lessons escaped most of the officers I met. *Why couldn't they see how violence projected violence, hate projected hate?* [Italics added]. . . .

"Jimmy," I said, "I am very sorry for you. The officer is sure you can't be trusted because you ran away . . . but I think you can. I know you ran away because of the bad things you let get the best of you."

And then I made it plain to Jimmy that however much I liked him I had been compelled to send him to the detention school—a mild name for the "kids'" jail, as it was known to Jimmy and his harum-scarum young friends.

---

[23] This is another good example of Lindsey's total commitment to his work.

He was penitent and a little later when he was alone with me the explanation came out through his tears.

"You see Judge," he said, "I was going to do just what you tolt me but on the way out there I passed that big field where the kids was playing ball. You know dhat's where our gang lives and, Gee whizz, I just couldn't pass dhe kids, I just couldn't, Judge. And before I knowed it I was up on my feet and I had ditched that street car. And then, when I remembered what you tolt me, I just got scared and I run home. And then, when the old man came home, I was under the bed scared to death, knowing he'd beat me up if he found me.

"I knowed I had missed my chance but I started for the street again when that fly cop comes along and pinches me on the spot. Gee, I thinks, what a fool I has been to t'row down dhe judge![24]

"The cop gives me a cussing and tells me he'll fix me dhis time. So he t'rows me in before I knows it and then I sees I ain't got no yell."

"I am glad you learned that lesson for yourself, Jimmy," I told him. "You think the cop wants to hurt you. But I hope you know I really believe that you can be trusted—I think you were just scared."

And, as in so many other cases, with this approach of tolerance and understanding, of confidence in the good rather than the evil there was in Jimmy, he rose magnificently to the occasion.

"Gee, Judge," he begged, "can't you give me another chance? Just give me the writ and I'll show 'em—I'll show 'em, Judge. I'll show that cop I can be trusted."[25]

"Of course you will, Jimmy," I answered, "I know you will."

---

[24] The appeal to loyalty to the Judge had taken apparently. Lindsey (1903) often emphasized his interdependence with his boys. He told them he was chancing his career on them, and they were chancing an unknown and likely tougher judge if he was forced to leave the bench.

[25] Lindsey sometimes appealed to the offenders' hostility to the law. As part of the "game of correction," Lindsey encouraged the youth to look upon his taking himself to reform school as a form of "fooling the cop" (Lindsey & Borough, 1931, p. 194).

How little I knew that it was the beginning of great events in a work that was to be known all over the world. Consciously or subconsciously, *I must have been a bit apprehensive* [italics added],[26] in those early days. For I stood at the window there alone in my chambers. I saw little Jimmy descend the courthouse steps—he too, alone—with his commitment papers in his own pocket—as he emerged from the great building out into the streets of the crowded city to join me in the great adventure of the "Dangerous Life."

True to his word, he braved all the temptation. He arrived alone. His fears had been conquered, his pride had triumphed. The papers were returned with "executed" in the small handwriting of little Jimmy: "Dear Judge, I am here—and I comes all by myself. Be sure and tell that cop" (Lindsey & Borough, 1931, pp. 166–170).[27]

It would be a mistake to believe that Lindsey relied only on such personal hypnotism to achieve his results. In one early instance, the police brought a chronic runaway into court, and called the newspapers to show up the "fool judge!" Lindsey still sent the boy to Golden, enlisting his aid in fooling both the police and the reporters. When the boy got to Golden, Lindsey heard that others, both grownups and children, had called him a "chump." Lindsey then went to Golden and told the boy's story before an assemblage of inmates and staff, praising the boy for his courage, loyalty, and self-control. Lindsey repeated this speech on innumerable occasions at Golden, in court, and in newspaper and magazine articles. He succeeded in changing the norm so that ". . . to 'ditch your paper and run', is a disgrace in Boyville now. A boy called on the Judge one day with an offer from the gang to 'lick' any kid that ditched his papers or in any other way went back on the Judge, and the Judge had some difficulty in explaining why that wasn't 'square' " (Steffens, 1909, p. 174). Lindsey saw to it that the very act of going to reform school became part of the culture of the group he

[26] This statement is a tribute either to Lindsey's defenses, or to his fearlessness, or to both!

[27] As part of his approach, Lindsey would give a boy paper and an envelope and ask him to write to him if he weakened, or when he arrived at the reform school. He stayed in contact with the boy.

was trying to help. His appeal to the "spark of the divine" was made in the context of helping the individual to meet the norms of his community, and in the context of their interdependence. Lindsey did not work with the individual alone but he worked with the entire community of which the boy, the judge, and the court were a part.

the institution of human relations

As part of his concern with helping children, some of Lindsey's later work was directed toward strengthening his Family Relations Court. Finding in many instances that the law protected property rights when it did not protect human rights, Lindsey succeeded in winning a number of reforms to protect the integrity of the family when the parents became involved with criminal matters, or when issues of non-support were involved. Lindsey attempted to establish informal procedures in a family court which would lead to a settlement of the case with a minimum of legal expense to the family and a minimum use of jail penalties to enforce support orders,[28] although he did fight for a law to make non-support a felony in Colorado. He also attempted to re-solve family disputes and to mediate in cases where divorce was contemplated. He would frequently meet with the contending parties in his chambers, dispensing with the services of lawyers, an action which won him the enmity of some members of the bar.

Lindsey actually was campaigning for a new social institution, a house of human welfare, or an institution of human relations,[29] which would take over some of the functions of civil, criminal, and divorce courts. He had in mind an institution to deal with illegitimacy, mental

[28] In our work with the Community Progress, Inc., Neighborhood Employment Centers (Sarason, et al., 1966) we recently encountered the case of a man who had been convicted of non-support. He spent sixty days in jail, lost his job, and gained a record which barred him from civil service employment, from employment in some security sensitive positions, and made him a criminal in the eyes of employers. How his family was served by this vengeful act of the law is far from clear.

[29] In 1914, before Healy published his book on the Individual Delinquent, Cincinnati established a Court of Domestic Relations which had exclusive jurisdiction over all cases involving children or the family. All divorce and alimony cases, all cases of juvenile delinquency, all cases of neglect, and all cases concerning the administration of mothers' pensions came to the one court. The court established a

or physical disease, divorce, non-support desertion, statutory rape, and similar social problems. The institution would be staffed by experts

central registry so that it had available all salient facts concerning individuals and families who had any contact with public or semi-public agencies in the city over the past few years. As part of the court organization, there were two psychologists and a psychiatrist, and there was a working relationship with the vocational bureau of the public school system and the Central Mental Hygiene Clinic. The director of the psychological clinic of the school's vocational bureau was a supervisor in the court clinic. A further interlocking relationship was described between the court and the Central Mental Hygiene Clinic and the Cincinnati General Hospital. There were intimate relationships with the Boarding Home Bureau, which provided foster homes for children needing special care, and with the Big Brothers organizations, which maintained paid directors and a staff of trained social workers to supervise children entrusted to their care. The Rotary and other civic and luncheon clubs assisted in caring for groups of both delinquent and dependent children.

> It has been tacitly, if not expressly, determined by the social agencies of Cincinnati, the public schools and all the civic organizations that no child manifesting symptoms of conduct disorders shall enter a criminal career (Hoffman, 1925, p. 259).

It became the policy of the court to send all delinquent children and others who needed special care and treatment to the clinic, and it permitted the directors of the clinic and the school authorities to prescribe treatment without the appearance of children in the court. The court supervised the work and used its powers of coercion when parents would not cooperate or when legal commitment was necessary. The court proposed and worked toward an ideal in which the public schools would take responsibility for caring for delinquent and pre-delinquent cases so that the stigma of criminality would not be placed upon them.

The Cincinnati Court tried to convert itself into an organization which referred cases for diagnosis and treatment to the organization, institution, or individual best qualified for the purpose. It saw itself as eliminating from the law hostility toward the lawbreaker and as substituting a social objective. It operated under the theory that the principle of retribution was unworkable and that a "kindly, sympathetic and helpful attitude toward those who fall is the only one that can possibly succeed, either in rehabilitating the individual or in protecting personal and property rights" (Hoffman, 1925, p. 263).

Judge Hoffman claimed that no girls had been committed to the State Industrial School for Girls from Cincinnati for the previous three years, and out of a population of 1,200 boys in the State Industrial School, only six were from Cincinnati. Official Juvenile Court hearings had practically ceased in Cincinnati. There is evidence that the Cincinnati system was at least as successful if not more than other juvenile courts of its day in preventing further delinquency (Sutherland & Cressey, 1960, pp. 412–413). Thomas and Thomas (1928), however, had a less positive view of the Cincinnati system, believing that its case work standards were poor, and that only a small number of cases were actually served through the court's clinical facilities.

The 1914 Cincinnati Domestic Relations Court presents another model which deserves renewed attention in this day and age of community mental health.

in problems of mental hygiene and by lawyers with backgrounds in biology, sociology, and psychology. It would be able to call upon the schools and social agencies as needed and would handle all such cases, even having the power to grant divorces when indicated.

As part of his concern for people, Lindsey at that time also favored the repeal of anti-birth control information laws. In his work, he came to understand that sexual ignorance created many problems, and he supported a bill which would enable school boards to provide courses in mental hygiene, in child rearing, in the art of marital relationships, and in sex. He believed such education should be mandatory for adults as well as for children. His total concept of prevention and treatment provides another service model for those concerned with community mental health (Lindsey, 1925; Lindsey & Evans, 1925; Lindsey & Borough, 1931).

change in Denver's Juvenile Court

From 1901 until the election of 1924, Lindsey was able to win election or appointment to the bench. In 1924, he won his office by only 300 votes, and in 1927, the Colorado Supreme Court found that in one district he carried there were fraudulent election practices of sufficient seriousness to warrant throwing out the results of that precinct. Lindsey was then removed from the bench. He claimed the Supreme Court was filled with political enemies, but even if he was right, that does not account for the very close election when in former times he had won by massive pluralities or he had been appointed to this office through the force of public sentiment.

Lindsey was a man of the reform era, but the 1920's was a period of great political conservatism. In Colorado in 1924, the KKK was at the height of its influence, as it was in a number of states. Total KKK membership was estimated at four-and-a-half million (Allen, 1959, p. 47). In Denver and throughout the state, flaming crosses were commonplace. Negroes, Jews, and Catholics were terrorized. KKK members were elected to school boards and made their way into the courts. A mayor of Denver and a senator of Colorado were reputed to be members. Lindsey writes of armed Klansmen entering his court while he was trying a Klan leader. Characteristically, in the 1924 campaign, Lindsey spoke out against the Klan and defended the persecuted minorities.

He also continued speaking out for his concept of companionate marriage. In urging repeal of anti-birth control information laws and in urging more realistic divorce laws, Lindsey won the opposition of the Catholic clergy, who attacked him en masse from their pulpits. Moreover, his enemies, not satisfied in ousting him, urged that his Juvenile Court also be abolished. The court was not abolished, but in Lindsey's place was appointed a judge who evidently did not follow Lindsey's policies. Lindsey tells of his feelings on leaving the court and at the same time gives us some insight into some of the reasons he could not perpetuate his work.

> In the days following the court ouster I walked the streets of Denver in a daze. At night I passed the court house, where for twenty-eight years I had carried on my work, looking up at its darkened rooms with unutterable yearning.
>
> In these rooms I had brought back to decency and citizenship thousands of boys and girls, saved from destruction thousands of homes, written dozens of items of legislation that, after years of struggle, had become part of the established laws not only in my own state but in many other states and in foreign countries.
>
> And as I looked I saw men, women, and children, with their deep, dark secrets and their wretchedness, again streaming up the stairs to those rooms. I know their desperate need of sympathy and understanding. . . . I heard the cry of those people for the bread of life, the artistry of love, the glowing technique of service, answered by the same cold formalism that I had driven from the court a quarter of a century before (Lindsey & Borough, 1931, pp. 10–11).

Lindsey's institution did not survive him in the form he created and it is important to ask why his procedure was not institutionalized so that it would continue. It is clear that his loss of popularity and political defeat were part of a conservative spirit which made it all but impossible for reformers to pursue any meaningful program. Lindsey was an outspoken reformer and his proposals for companionate marriage and for an institution of human welfare were proposals for reforms in two of the basic institutions of society, the courts and marriage. The temper of the times no longer permitted one to take liberties with basic social institutions.

the "routinization of charisma"

The concept of a juvenile court spread throughout the nation and throughout the world (Addams, 1925, pp. 267–273). However, Lindsey's clinical contributions were lost. His life's work, as he so poignantly says, "turned into a mockery."

To some extent, Lindsey's was the triumph and the failure of charisma. He could in his own person gain the affection and sympathy of thousands of youth, but he was unable to institutionalize his own practice. He left neither a trained successor nor a corps of dedicated followers who would practice his approach to rehabilitation through the courts. When Lindsey left the Colorado bench his probation officers, who were his appointees, also left the court. The system did not permit him to perpetuate his practices.

His legal works gained widespread recognition, but he left no comparable body of technical and theoretical writings which could be used as the basis for institutionalizing his practices. The description of the Saturday morning report sessions, for example, appear only in the 1904 report, and are not mentioned to any significant extent in the 1931 book. Most of the descriptions of his work appear in popular sources, and as far as we have been able to tell, his clinical work was never regarded with any degree of seriousness by mental health professionals. Perhaps their professionalism and emphasis on psychoanalytic theory and psychotherapeutic practice may have been a reason Lindsey's innovations were ignored. In as important a survey of clinical practices in the United States as *The Child in America* (Thomas & Thomas, 1928), Lindsey is mentioned only because he organized classes in which widowed mothers receiving pensions could discuss the problems of their children.

In part, Lindsey's personality must have been responsible for a failure to win adherents. He approached many problems with a head-on assault guaranteed to create opposition. In some respects he reminds one of an Old Testament prophet who spoke out against wickedness and hypocrisy and found that his message brought him vituperation and calumny.

Lindsey's personality seems to reflect characteristics of his father and his grandfather, both men of integrity who did not fear standing up for what they believed. From his early days in school, Lindsey did not hesitate to speak out. Perhaps his situation as a Catholic in a Baptist community led him to develop his particular style. Lindsey's aristocratic background and his personal experience of poverty and hardship may have given him the range of experience which enabled him to relate with the very poor and with those in positions of wealth and power.

However, in some respects Lindsey seemed to be an impulsive, irascible character, given to high-handed actions. A newspaper carried a story of another court reversing one of his decisions in a paternity case. The judge in the appeals court felt Lindsey had acted to promote a wedding on very little grounds. In another instance, Lindsey physically attacked a man who had falsely accused him of improprieties with children. The attack took place in court during the trial of a libel suit which Lindsey won. Lindsey seemed to enjoy being the center of turmoil, and sometimes, as in the episode in which he was ejected from a church for shouting at a bishop, others questioned his lack of dignity if not of judgment. It is unquestionably true that he stirred strong feelings in people. When we visited Denver in 1966, one old timer cursed when we inquired about Lindsey. A respected professional who knew him well said that he thought the Judge was "a little crazy." Other people remembered some of his rehabilitation schemes as half-baked and told of instances in which his efforts to use people in the community to help children backfired and hurt the people involved. The same man who could write legal history could endorse a safety razor in magazine ads, and knowingly or unknowingly, have his mother appear in widow's weeds to talk for him at a political rally which threatened to go badly for him. Lindsey was obviously a complex personality who both attracted and repulsed others. To what extent his individual style, like Witmer's, caused others to take him less seriously than they might is an open question.

Lindsey lived to see the bare outlines of his concept preserved in institutional form, but he could not guarantee that he himself would be reproduced. In the process of institutionalizing an innovation, in "routinizing charisma," as Max Weber (1964) puts it, either positions within an institution are filled by those who lack the appropriate human qualities or the positions themselves are so bureaucratized that initiative and flexibility are lost. The experiences in Chicago and in Denver suggest that although the innovators were aware that certain human qualities were essential for work with youth in the Juvenile Court, the innovators were powerless to guarantee that people with the necessary qualities would be attracted to the work and, if attracted, would be permitted to function as their instincts dictated.

The activities which were at the heart of Lindsey's work, the deep involvement with the community and the effort to make the court the agent of the youth it served, would today be denied to publicly supported probation workers. Certainly reform would never become the concern of judges who rotate through a low prestige institution (Polier, 1964). In the last twenty years, one would be hard pressed to find examples of juvenile court personnel who challenged slumlords, who fought for recreational facilities, who attacked inequities in job opportunity, who pressed for better school facilities, who fought for the rights of families on welfare, or who attacked political failure to provide adequate resources for dealing with human problems. The lack of facilities for residential care of neglected children and the lack of treatment and rehabilitative facilities for disturbed youth have plagued the courts for years, but there is little evidence that Juvenile Court personnel have been involved in the battle for reform.

The present day mental health professional, the psychiatrist, the social worker, the clinical psychologist attached to a court would not view it as part of his professional function to change the situation. The present day professional seeks to help the individual to change himself. At a recent conference on the Juvenile Court, the best solution the psychiatrist on the panel could present was an increase in group therapy. The present day professional seems not to have faith that each individual contains a "spark of the divine" and he does not see it as his function to help create the conditions under which growth can occur. The mental health professional operates with a treatment orientation which separates his patient and himself from involvement with the broader society of which they both are a part. It is paradoxical that any mental health professional who acted in the tradition of a Jane Addams or a Ben Lindsey would be viewed as acting in an untraditional manner indeed, so far have we as mental health professionals forgotten our origins.

10

the child guidance clinic—
a product of the 1920's

The next major service to develop after the juvenile court was the community child guidance clinic. It began in the period following the First World War, a time when reform sentiment was dead. The development of the child guidance clinic provides a contrast with the forms developed over the previous thirty years.

In 1921, the Commonwealth Fund launched a bold program for the prevention of juvenile delinquency. As part of that program, demonstration child guidance clinics were established in a number of cities. Our contemporary privately supported community child guidance clinics developed out of these models. The child guidance clinic, as originally conceptualized in the Commonwealth Fund's program, was meant to be a vital force in the community, closely interrelated with a variety of other agencies and the schools, and designed to influence them. In today's terms the Commonwealth program would be a community mental health program. However, the clinics rather quickly adopted their modern form. From agencies with a mission to modify aspects of the community, and to provide a preventive service, the clinics became treatment agencies, dealing with individuals who came seeking help. This change from conception to practice took place in a certain social and professional context, and an examination of the process of change will provide illumination of the forces shaping mental health practices.

the 1920's

To understand the child guidance clinic, it is necessary to look at the decade in which it developed, the ten years following World War I that has come to be known as the "Roaring Twenties." World War I had focused America's attention on an external enemy. The problems of the cities, of immigrants, of poverty, of social welfare, and of social reform, all of which concerned the previous generation, were put aside as the nation dedicated itself to making the world "safe for democracy." In the post-war period the reform movement never regained momentum, for the mood of the nation had changed and so had the problems which occupied its attention (Goldman, 1956; Schlesinger, 1957; Allen, 1959). Despite some fairly radical shifts in the role of women, and despite some change in sexual mores, the decade of the 1920's was basically conservative in a political and a social sense. It was the age of Babbitts.

From 1920 until the Great Depression, liberals and social reformers were without power or influence. The First World War promoted a belief in the rightness of the American way of life and fostered an almost fanatic demand for 100 percent Americanism. The phrase "splendid isolation" and the rejection of the League of Nations characterize the feeling of the times. The Bolshevik revolution frightened the nation, and the reaction against liberalism and foreigners was pronounced. New Year's Day of 1920 saw the Palmer raids in which 6,000 "Reds" were arrested. Professors suspected of radicalism were threatened with dismissal; schoolteachers were forced to sign loyalty oaths; those with unorthodox political, social, or economic ideas learned to keep quiet. Before and during the war many social workers had flirted with socialistic concepts and had been active in pacifist and anti-war movements. When after the war patriotic societies sprang up to point out the menaces to America, liberal civic and welfare agencies were favorite targets (Holden, 1922; Linn, 1935; Duffus, 1938). The oppressive atmosphere of the day led to an unrelieved conformity of ideas which stifled liberal reform.

The demand for 100 percent Americanism was manifested in a series of restrictive immigration bills. In 1921, in 1924, and again in 1927, Congress passed laws making it increasingly difficult for immigrants from Southern and Eastern Europe to enter this country. National, racial, and religious prejudices were aroused and intolerance flared. Some of the most vicious of race riots occurred in the early 1920's, and the Ku Klux Klan found fertile soil for its growth. By 1924, its membership was estimated at four and one half million; it had political power throughout the country and not only in the South, for its terror even touched New York City. To be sure, despite the business prosperity, there was still poverty with its attendant disorganization and misery, but little attention was paid to it. Even the labor unions had taken a conservative turn (Bernstein, 1966). In such a social context, the major portion of the public mind would listen to and support only those who asserted that this was indeed the best of all possible worlds, and it looked with suspicion and hostility upon those who said differently. It was in this climate that the radicals Sacco and Vanzetti could be tried, executed, and forgotten.

The decade of the 1920's was the businessman's era. Beginning with Harding and continuing with Coolidge and Hoover, conservative business interests found strong support in the White House. Harding called for a return to "normalcy"; Coolidge said, "The chief business of the American people is business." The courts, the regulatory agencies, and the legislatures all supported business, and indeed there was an almost unprecedented period of sustained economic growth and prosperity. The businessman was revered, the millionaire was an idol and an ideal. Throughout the decade it was the individual hero, a Lindbergh, a Babe Ruth, a movie star, or even an Al Capone who could capture public attention and admiration. The tenets of conservative Darwinism had revived, and keen, even cutthroat competition was the order of the day. If a man failed in the prosperous world of the 1920's, it was because he lacked something inside himself. The emphasis on self-help, on the individual willing himself to success, is symbolized in Emil Coué's aphorism, "Day by day, in every way, I am getting better and better." Coué, as popular as Mah Jong and the crossword puzzle, captivated audiences across the nation.

While pressures toward social and economic reform were minimal in the 1920's, reform in "manners and morals" (Allen, 1959), that is, reform in personal codes and personal values, was pronounced. Such changes were in keeping with the emphasis on self-development.

When the Nineteenth Amendment to the Constitution was ratified in 1920, assuring women the right to vote, it was a major event, but only one manifestation of the progress women were making in their long battle to achieve equal status with men. The role of women was undergoing drastic change. During World War I their labor was solicited, and many continued to work even after "the boys came marching home." Appliances and canned and processed foods began to free them from the kitchens. Concomitant with the increasing independence of women and the prosperous times, there was a drastic rise in the divorce rate.

The virtues of pre-marital chastity and marital fidelity were open to question as never before, and in some instances adulterous affairs were undertaken not secretly, but as a matter of living out a modern value. Lindsey's (Lindsey & Evans, 1925) proposals for companionate marriage were timely, but the violent reaction to formal proposals for a change in the marital institution suggests a strong underlying anxiety about the changes which were occurring.

The erosion of the sexual double standard was manifested by women, especially the young, flinging off corsets, donning short skirts, using cosmetics boldly, and dancing even more boldly to the good jazz that was served with the bad liquor they drank in the speakeasies. Open discussion of sex and free love was the order of the day. Sex movies, sex magazines, and confession magazines reached millions. Automobiles gave the young travelling bedrooms free from parental surveillance. Prohibition did not prohibit, but added spice to the adventure of crossing forbidden limits (Lindsey & Evans, 1925; Lynd & Lynd, 1929; Allen, 1959).

The 1920's was the decade in which psychoanalysis took hold in the United States, and to some extent, it was psychoanalytic thinking which provided an intellectual, scientific rationale for the changes. Popular psychoanalysis, emphasizing the free expression of sexual impulse and the danger of "frustration," filled magazines and books and was a principal topic of conversation in some circles. It is said that almost everyone who was anyone in the Greenwich Village set was in analysis. Psychoanalysis as a modern science was eagerly accepted among those for whom the older religious and moral symbols had grown stale, although as a discipline, it was not yet entrenched in the medical schools (Brill, 1939; Burgess, 1939).

Given the marked changes in manners and morals, it was no

wonder that parents felt uncertainty about what was right. To add to their uncertainty, popular magazines, Sunday supplements, and even radio, reaching millions, brought word of the change and advice about how to live in the modern world. The advice was as conflicting then as it is now. Popular Freud, popular Watson (Watson, 1928), and popular Gesell (Gesell, 1928) were widely disseminated. Don't frustrate your child, train him to be what you want; he's in a stage of life, he'll grow out of it; breast feed, don't breast feed; punish, don't punish; sex education, no sex education; your child will grow up to be a neurotic. And of course, tradition was not without its defenders. It is little wonder that the child guidance clinics, as specialized facilities offering expertise in an ambiguous area, met popular needs and flourished. Cross (1934) felt child guidance to be one of the "well defined social movements of our time."

The 1920's then, represented a period of strong social and political conservatism, in which the problems stemming from the societal order were neglected or ignored. It was also a period in which apparent opportunity for the individual was great, if the individual was able to play the game. If one didn't succeed in life, it was one's own fault. Moreover, there was a gross attack on certain traditions and a marked shift in sexual attitudes and in the female role. The changes created a general uncertainty and a search on the part of individuals for new values around which to organize one's life. Science was the new god, and the psychiatrists, psychologists, psychoanalysts, and social workers were his disciples. It was in this social context with its emphasis on the individual, an emphasis consistent with the psychoanalytic view of man, that the child guidance clinics developed.

the Commonwealth Fund's Program for the Prevention of Delinquency

Although the child guidance movement developed rapidly[1] in the 1920's, the program initiated by the Commonwealth Fund involving but seven

---

[1] Lowrey and Smith (1933) estimate that in 1921 there were but seven clinics showing the characteristic child guidance structure; the number grew to 102 by 1927. Further data on the growth of community clinics may be found in Stevenson and Smith (1934). H. Witmer (1940) presents similar data showing the growth of state-supported clinics for the same period.

clinics was highly influential in shaping the direction of that growth. The pattern of the privately supported community child guidance clinic with the now traditional team consisting of psychiatrist, social worker, and psychologist was set by the experience of the demonstration clinics. Two of the agencies established by the Commonwealth Fund, the Bureau of Children's Guidance (Lee & Kenworthy, 1929) and the Institute for Child Guidance (Lowrey & Smith, 1933), were prime training centers in the fields of child psychiatry and psychiatric social work, and to a lesser extent in clinical psychology. In addition, some of the other demonstration clinics also served as training agencies from their inception. Thus, the Commonwealth Fund's program not only presented model clinics, but as training centers, the clinics helped to influence thinking and practice throughout the country.

David Levy, one of the leading figures in American child psychiatry, has said:

> The name[2] and the formula of "child guidance" were stamped firmly on the history of psychiatry by the philanthropic and administrative support of the Commonwealth Fund. A five-year period of demonstration clinics throughout the country was, in a way, one of the most successful enterprises in the field of philanthropy when judged by a criterion used by a number of philanthropic foundations, that a project proves its worth when it is taken over and supported by the community. In that sense, the demonstration clinics were most successful. Since they were first launched, about 30 years ago, over 200 child guidance clinics have been established and supported by local agencies in these United States (Levy, 1952).

Because of the great influence of the Commonwealth Fund clinics, it is most useful to focus on their development rather than on other

---

[2] E. K. Wickman, psychologist, and Mildred Scoville, social worker, members of the very earliest demonstration clinic teams, coined the name "child guidance." Wickman (personal communication) recalls that he and Scoville were looking for a name which would avoid the stigma associated with the label "psychiatry," a label which then meant a profession dealing with crazy people who were locked up. They settled on "child guidance clinic," a variation of the name of the earlier established Bureau of Children's Guidance.

clinics which developed at the same time. Although the Commonwealth Fund obviously did not establish or dictate the pattern of service in all of the developing clinics, nonetheless the experience of these clinics was undoubtedly critical in that era.

A few words are in order about the Commonwealth Fund, which provided the basic financial support for the demonstration clinics. The Commonwealth Fund was established in 1918 by Mrs. Stephen V. Harkness "to do something for the welfare of mankind" (Commonwealth Fund, 1963). The Fund reflected the ideals and practices of the previous twenty-five years. In the latter part of the 19th century, men who made great fortunes from the massive industrial growth of the post-Civil War period developed a humanistic concern which was manifested in lavish contributions toward social betterment. As background to this new concern we may note that religious leaders (Hopkins, 1940; Abell, 1943) decried the business ethics of the period and urged a more Christian approach to human problems. Moreover, there was pressure for the relief of social problems and there was talk of the reduction of inequality through the redistribution of income. Even the shocking notion of an income tax had begun to be bruited about. The Beards (1927) speculate about other motives which guided the philanthropy of the day, but beyond the motives, philanthropy after the 1890's turned its attention toward the prevention of human misery by attacking its basic social causes. The focus of attack shifted from individual charity to massive social work, but not in the casework sense. Rather, it was in the sense of contributing to an assault on sickness and misery by supporting the humanities and the sciences and by stimulating community planning to solve the problems of the day.

It was in such a tradition that the Commonwealth Fund developed its first major undertaking in the field of health and welfare, the Program for the Prevention of Juvenile Delinquency. The name and the intent to focus on delinquency reveals in the planning of the program the premise that the social climate of the immediate past with its emphasis on broad social reform would continue in the immediate future. It is no criticism of the group which planned the program that they could not foresee the future. However, it is clear that the problem of helping children was approached with a limited appreciation of the broader social forces which had brought the problem of delinquency to the forefront of concern earlier. In the decade to come, other forces arose to shape clinical interests and practices.

The Commonwealth Program involved the cooperative effort of the New York School of Social Work, of the National Committee for Mental Hygiene's Division on the Prevention of Delinquency, and the National Committee on Visiting Teachers. In addition, a Joint Committee on Methods of Preventing Delinquency was organized specifically to act both as coordinator and publicist for this program.

The Commonwealth Fund's program, while important in promoting the growth of clinics throughout the country, was not a truly innovative program in the sense that it never intentionally created a new form of help. The program was designed to spread already developed forms of help. The New York School of Social Work was given funds for a clinic to encourage the training of psychiatric social workers, visiting teachers, and probation officers. As we have seen, probation officers were part of the Juvenile Court, an agency developed some twenty years earlier and past its heyday. The visiting teacher movement had also developed some fifteen years earlier. By 1921, it was well established as part of the New York public school system and others as well.

Formal training in psychiatric social work was an outgrowth of the demand for help for soldiers suffering from emotional shock. The first training center for psychiatric social workers had already opened at Smith College in the summer of 1918 and courses in mental hygiene and in psychiatry had been available to social work students at the New York School since 1917.

By 1921, Witmer's clinic was a quarter of a century old. Healy had left the Juvenile Psychopathic Institute (by now the Institute for Juvenile Research) in Chicago to Herman Adler and had gone to Boston to establish the Judge Baker Center. By 1914 psychological clinics were numerous enough to provide the material for a comprehensive review (Smith, 1914).

The models which were supported were already in existence when the Commonwealth Fund's program developed. This is not to take away from the significance of the program, but simply to reinforce the statement that the model which was to be propagated in the 1920's was a model developed in the previous generation. The Fund intended to direct its efforts to adding to the resources readily available to the field (Commonwealth Fund, 1921–1922).

The demonstration clinics were to be developed under the auspices of the National Committee for Mental Hygiene's Division on the Prevention of Delinquency.[3] The National Committee itself was a product of the earlier period of reform, the creation of Clifford Beers, founder of the mental hygiene movement. His book, *A Mind That Found Itself* (Beers, 1908), had a profound influence on humanizing the care of the mentally ill in hospitals. In 1909, with the active support of William James and many psychiatrists and philanthropists, he founded the National Committee for Mental Hygiene. The National Committee was at first concerned with humanizing patient care, but it soon turned its attention to the problem of the prevention of disorder. As a consequence of its activities, psychopathic wards were developed in city hospitals (Southard, 1914) to provide first aid for mental patients; outpatient clinics were developed to deal with incipient mental illness (Abelson, 1966); special programs for training the mentally deficient for a place in society were supported; and there was much political and public relations activity designed to spread the concepts of mental hygiene (Barker, 1918; Cross, 1934).

As the concept of prevention became prevalent, and as the new psychology became accepted, the roots of mental disorder were traced further and further back into childhood. By 1921, psychoanalytic thinking and its derivatives had begun to pervade the fields of psychiatry, social work, and child care. It was only natural then that the National Committee would become interested in a program to help children, since help in childhood was seen as a primary means of preventing mental disorder and criminality in adulthood.

In January of 1921, the Commonwealth Fund and the National Committee sponsored a conference of an advisory committee to draw up guidelines for the Commonwealth Fund's program to prevent delinquency. Among others who attended this conference in Lakewood, New Jersey, were William Healy, Augusta Bronner, and Charles W. Hoffman, judge of Cincinnati's Juvenile and Domestic Relations Court. Included were representatives of psychiatry, education, and social work.

The concepts of prevention which guided the development of the demonstration clinics may be gleaned from the following excerpts from

[3] The Division on the Prevention of Delinquency was formed after a representative of the Commonwealth Fund approached the National Committee to ascertain its interest in the Commonwealth Fund's program. The National Committee showed its interest by forming a division of delinquency within its organization. The influence of the availability of funds on the problems which are studied and treated is brought out here (Stevenson, 1948).

the conference's recommendations (Stevenson, 1948, pp. 53–56) :*

> It is our opinion that lack of knowledge by teachers and school authorities of existing information regarding disorders of conduct result in many instances in the actual causation of delinquency through mismanagement of incipient disorders of this kind and, to a much greater extent, in failure to carry out preventive measures in an environment presenting many favorable opportunities. . . .
>
> It is our opinion that certain agencies created for the express purpose of protecting, training, and caring for children not only fail in many instances to prevent delinquency, on account of their poorly trained personnel and the inadequate social, psychological, and medical diagnoses on children coming under their care, but through improper methods of management and institutional administration, actually contribute to the production of delinquency in those exposed to such unfavorable conditions. . . .
>
> It is our opinion that . . . through mismanagement of their mental handicap and the lack of proper facilities for dealing with feeblemindedness in its institutional, educational, and community aspects, [many] needlessly become delinquents.
>
> It is our opinion that attainment of the general aims of the social hygiene organization will tend to reduce delinquency and that a relationship exists between sex education and delinquency which requires careful study in order to determine the efficiency of sex education and the specific methods by which it is carried on.
>
> It is our opinion that all children should have opportunities for the use of spare time in ways that, on the one hand, are not harmful to the community and, on the other, give to the children themselves opportunities for self-expression and a satisfying sense of physical and social achievement.

It was recommended that agencies providing suitable recreational facilities and opportunities be encouraged by generous support.

---

*Copyright, American Orthopsychiatric Association, Inc., reproduced by permission.

> It is our opinion that the participation of children in certain
> industries, such as street trades, home work, and such sea-
> sonal trades as canning and berrying, increase delinquency.

The opinions and recommendations called for the expansion of the
work of the Juvenile and Family Relations Courts, the further development of probation procedures, and the reform of the detention homes
associated with Juvenile Courts and the training and reform schools.

A further excerpt from the conference report gives the reader an
idea of its strong reform sentiment.

> While the implication of some of the foregoing conclusions
> is that certain agencies created and maintained for the ex-
> press purpose of safeguarding childhood, and in some in-
> stances of dealing specifically with juvenile delinquency
> have not succeeded in making full use of their opportunities
> and through unfortunate conditions growing out of their
> work, sometimes even tend to increase delinquency, the
> opinions expressed are set forth for the purpose of directing
> attention to the importance of correcting specific defects and
> not with any idea of destructive criticism of activities which
> were instituted for high humanitarian purposes. . . . We be-
> lieve that social agencies created for humanitarian purposes
> can properly be examined . . . and that the results of such
> examination are certain to be [as] beneficial (Stevenson,
> 1948, p. 56).

The tone is not impassioned, but the message is clearly social
reform to be achieved by changing existing social organizations. The
report closes with a recommendation for the training of medical, psychological, and social service personnel to carry out the work of diagnosis and to disseminate modern scientific information concerning conduct disorders and the principles which underlie their treatment and
prevention. The education of others who had primary responsibility for
the care of children who might become delinquent was to be accomplished by their participation in case studies. This was viewed as the
major function of any new clinical service.[4]

---

[4] It is noteworthy that the group organizing the clinics viewed social change as the
inevitable result of education; that is, of acquainting people with facts. Their views
are similar to those originally entertained by the settlement workers in their quest
for social change.

Two concepts employed in this report are worth underlining. First, the report adopts a situational orientation, arguing that it is the institution and the social setting which are largely responsible for problems, and that it is the institutional or the social setting which should be altered in order to permit the individual to grow. Second, in emphasizing the importance of the institutional setting, the report recommends that professional services be directed toward educating and helping the institutions to carry out their work. There does not seem to be any thought at this time that the professional mental health worker should establish an institution which would treat in its own right. There is no statement that what is needed is a treatment facility which would be relatively isolated from the community, but rather the objective was to put the professional mental health worker in ever closer touch with the community setting so that he could influence it. The later development of the child guidance clinic has to be considered in light of the philosophy expressed in this conference report.[5]

It is our viewpoint that the thinking reflected in the Lakewood conference was the thinking of the pre-World War I period. The conceptions underlying the development of the clinics and the objectives for the clinics reflect the viewpoint of the social reformer and focus on

---

[5] The following statement by Herman M. Adler, Healy's successor as director of the Institute for Juvenile Research in Chicago clearly indicates that the viewpoint expressed by the participants in the Lakewood Conference was not peculiar to that particular group:

> The outstanding fact, however, of this whole discussion is that the psychopathologist and the physician are coming into closer contact with social problems than ever before; and that as society is becoming more intergrated [sic] so the psychopathologist is becoming more specialized, and psychiatry must concern itself more and more with the social aspects as manifested in human behavior and therefore must work in greater harmony than ever before with psychologists, teachers, economists and sociologists (Adler, 1922, pp. 19–20).

Adler's viewpoint is important because his institute was one of the first if not the only center in the pre-World War I period in which training in child psychiatry and in child guidance was available (Levy, 1952).

A similar statement, particularly with respect to the schools, may be found in Campbell's (1918) paper discussing the results of a survey of the mental health problems of Baltimore school children. Campbell felt that not necessarily the psychiatrist but the educational process, the schools, the visiting teacher, the psychiatrically oriented school nurse, and the school physician would be the prime therapeutic agents.

institutional change, but the period of the 1920's was no longer an era in which the call for institutional change would be heeded. It is our thesis that the later development of the clinics was shaped by the spirit of the 1920's, a spirit which would support individual treatment and be hostile to institutional change. We shall try to trace some of the social and professional forces which resulted in changes in objectives and practice in the child guidance clinics.

the medical model versus applied sociology

It was obvious from the very beginning that the medical model of treating the sick who would be brought to the clinic was inadequate to the task of truly serving a community. Surveys and the early experience of the clinics suggested the impossibility of serving any but the tiniest fraction of cases. A survey conducted by the National Committee for Mental Hygiene in Cincinnati in 1921 found that two out of three who came before the Juvenile Court were mentally abnormal, that 13 percent of the public school population deviated from normal mental health, and that 6 percent of the public school population showed conduct disorders sufficiently severe to repeatedly bring themselves to the authorities' attention (Stevenson, 1948).

One of the very first activities of the Division on the Prevention of Delinquency was to supervise a mental hygiene clinic in Monmouth County, New Jersey, in 1922. The clinic was sponsored by the Laura Spellman Rockefeller Fund. Although it limited its scope to diagnostic work, the task was too large for a full-time clinic in a county of 100,000. In the second year of its operation, the clinic modified its procedures to serve three communities within the county. "*Nevertheless, within three months a waiting list of 200 existed. This emphasized the immensity of the task of child guidance and the impossibility of securing coverage by direct service in any community. It showed the necessity of adapting clinical processes for indirect service* [italics added]" (Stevenson, 1948, p. 64).

In 1921, according to Stevenson (1948), helping a child meant that the mental health professional team make an accurate medical, social, and psychological diagnosis and transmit scientific findings to personnel in the agency which referred the child. The belief was that once others had been shown the "truth" about the child and had received recommendations about how to handle the problem, the referring agency would be served, and would then, in most cases, carry out the treatment. The planning group for the Commonwealth program had recognized the institutional contribution to the problem of delinquency. The answer to the institutional problem was to change the institution by educating personnel to think in a mental health framework. The case was to be the medium of education. Hopefully, the proper training of more psychiatric social workers, of more probation officers, and of more visiting teachers would make the problem easier, and, indeed, an important part of the Commonwealth program included the development and support of training programs. However, the essence of the professional approach was to remain in close contact with the referring source in order to facilitate treatment and educate the referring source.

By the time the actual plans for the program were drawn up, about a year after the Lakewood Conference, the goals had already shifted from the reform of institutions and social agencies to a concern with prevention on a clinical level. Prevention, in the report drawn by Barry C. Smith, a trained social worker who was general director of the Commonwealth Fund, meant the prevention of further difficulty for an individual who had already come to the attention of some helping service (Commonwealth Fund, 1922). By the time the first demonstration clinic started, the workers did not feel that reform of social agencies was their primary professional concern. Rather they felt their first professional responsibility was a thorough examination of the child and the development of a treatment plan for the agency responsible for the child.

Since the early workers felt that factual knowledge of the child would inevitably lead to better treatment by the responsible agencies, there was little thought given to the problem of gaining the cooperation of various agencies in carrying out treatment plans. By the time the clinics started to function, either by design or because the climate of the times militated against far-reaching reforms, the focus was upon the individual child rather than on stimulating change in agencies (E. K. Wickman, personal communication). This shift in viewpoint presaged an ever greater emphasis on treatment centered within the confines of a therapy room, with the consequent isolation of the clinics from other agencies.

the organization of the early child guidance clinics

Although the clinics began with a staff of a psychiatrist, a psychologist, and one or more psychiatric social workers, the organization and functioning of the clinics in the early days differed from those today. In this section we will describe two clinics, one in Minneapolis and one in Cleveland, and their varied functions.

They started with similar staffs and both of these demonstration clinics set a pattern for service which was continued when permanent clinics were established. For our purposes, it is the variety of staffing and consultation arrangements which is of interest.

The staff of the clinic in the Twin Cities (Minneapolis and St. Paul) demonstration consisted of a psychiatrist, three fellows in psychiatry, two psychologists, six social workers, and social work students. The clinic developed a loaned-worker system in which thirty-nine social workers from several of the local agencies spent periods up to three months as members of the clinic staff, participating in casework under supervision. The purpose of the system was to help the agency workers meet the problems on their own and at the same time to familiarize the agencies with the services the clinic could offer (Stevenson & Smith, 1934).

Particularly close relationships were developed with the Minneapolis public schools, which had a large staff of visiting teachers. When the demonstration clinic became a permanent facility, as a consequence of complex conflict with other agencies in the city, it was finally financed by the Board of Education. Its services, however, were available to the entire community. The clinic was housed in a children's hospital, which also had a school attached to it. The staff of twenty visiting teachers and ten speech teachers worked with clinic cases after they had been evaluated through the clinic. The three psychiatric social workers with the permanent clinic all had had experience as teachers, undoubtedly facilitating the relationship of the school to the clinic (Blanton, 1925; Stevenson, 1948).

The demonstration clinic established itself as an educational institution and the staff participated in a variety of educational ventures through the University of Minnesota. In addition to specific training offered to psychiatrists, social workers, and psychologists, the clinic staff participated in courses for social workers and teachers and offered courses in psychiatry in the medical school and courses in behavior problems in the department of education. There were additional seminars and lectures in the school of social work. As one outgrowth of the clinic's work, the state financed a rural demonstration clinic in mental hygiene under the direction of Dr. George Stevenson (Stevenson & Smith, 1934; Stevenson, 1948).

When the clinic became part of the public school system, the educational efforts continued. An elective course in mental hygiene was offered for high school juniors and seniors. Students in the course were asked to write life histories and those who indicated a need for advice were interviewed personally (Blanton, 1925). A course in mental hygiene was also offered for teachers and for parents.

A preventive service evolved through a behavior clinic established in the kindergartens. A behavior chart was developed, to be filled out by the kindergarten teacher for each child. When the charts indicated potential problems, parents were invited to discuss the situation with the social worker.

The demonstration clinic staff pioneered the open case conference as a teaching device, which was continued in the permanent clinic. Staff meetings in the permanent clinic were attended by the clinic staff, the child's teacher, the principal of the school, the visiting teacher, and any other social worker who wished to attend. The purpose of the open case conference is expressed in the following statement:

> Through discussion at this staff meeting, we hope that we may change the attitude of the teacher towards this child and towards all other children in her care, and the attitude of the principal towards her teachers and the children in the school. We hope that the teacher may stop thinking about behavior difficulties as unit characteristics, or as a moral obloquy, and think of the behavior of the child as symptomatic of some underlying cause. After the staff meeting we talk over the whole thing with the parents and try to change their attitude. We give them specific instructions about the training of the child and the social worker goes into the home from time to time to help carry out the program suggested (Blanton, 1925, pp. 99–100).

The service's preventive nature and the thinking of the participants is revealed:

In conclusion then, we believe that a mental hygiene clinic in the schools and colleges should be an integral part of the educational system, and it should not care for just those serious difficulties that might be referred by teacher or professor, but should reach all the children and students. In short, such a clinic should be a center for the education of the emotional life and for the understanding of the individual's own emotional reactions that make for success or failure. Such a clinic would be really a clinic of preventive medicine; a clinic in mental hygiene in the highest sense of the word (Blanton, 1925, p. 101).

The Cleveland demonstration clinic began in a city where social services and some psychiatric services were available, but it was the explicit purpose of the Cleveland demonstration to build the mental hygiene capacities of other agencies to the utmost.

The program of cooperative treatment was strongly developed. When a child was referred to the clinic by an agency, the agency social worker would make a special social examination, in consultation with the clinic's psychiatric social worker, and would have responsibility for carrying through the social treatment. The referring agency thus kept responsibility for treatment and agency workers hopefully acquired facility in dealing with other cases requiring a similar approach. Stevenson (1948) quotes from a report describing how agency workers used the clinic services as part of cooperative treatment:

All of the agencies with which we worked were most cooperative. Many of the workers fell into the habit of coming daily to the clinic to discuss various problems that had developed in their cases. For instance, here is a note in one case of a conversation between the social worker of the clinic and the probation officer: "Tommy bunked out again last night and his foster mother is terribly concerned. What do you think we'd better do? Shall I bring him in for another talk with the doctor? That last talk really impressed Tommy you know." Consequently, Tommy's case was thoroughly discussed, the foster home situation reviewed to date, and plans laid accordingly. Again quoting from notes on another case: "At last I have got Edna interested in try-

ing to learn something, but now she is determined to be a
stenographer. Do you think she's got brains enough?" The
clinic worker reviewed the vocational possibilities for Edna
in the light of the psychologist's report, and it was decided
to try to divert her ambitions to dressmaking or millinery
(Stevenson, 1948, p. 61).

Similar consultation services were provided to the Juvenile Court
and to agencies responsible for child welfare and for foster home care.
The demonstration clinic supplied a psychiatrist for a summer camp
for children with behavior problems and personality disturbances. In
another instance, consultation on weekends was offered for camp counselors at a normal summer camp. A variety of other services of a similar nature were provided to residential treatment homes and in later
years the clinic helped other agencies revamp their programs. The clinic
also took a leading role in establishing the Cleveland Mental Hygiene
Society because of its interest in preventive work. Many lectures were
given to community organizations. The staff of the clinic was intimately
engaged in the education of nurses and social workers and when there
was a school of education at the local university, instruction in child
guidance was offered to prospective teachers (Schumacher, 1948).

It is clear from these descriptions that some of the early clinics
were intimately involved in the community, that they made efforts to
help community agencies handle their mental hygiene problems, that
there was a distinct preventive orientation, and that they saw it as part
of their function to instill a mental hygiene viewpoint in those who
would have responsibility for the care of children.

However, as Schumacher (1948) points out, over the years the
clinics saw more and more children for full study and treatment and
decided they could not proceed satisfactorily without full control over
the case. While cooperative services and consultative services could be
helpful, the clinics felt that if the child required psychiatric treatment,
they must carry it out. Wickman (personal communication) who
worked in clinics in St. Louis, Dallas, Minneapolis, and Cleveland, noted
that the practice of treating patients in the clinic increased steadily from
1922 to 1928. To some extent, in Cleveland and elsewhere, it appears
as if the depression of the 1930's contributed the death blow to such
services because the agencies no longer had the funds to hire consultants.
However, the fact is that the earlier efforts to influence community

agencies were lost in the preference for full control over the treatment of a case, even though it was obvious that direct treatment could not serve social needs. What were the factors leading to changes in clinical practices?

training and child guidance

While it is undoubtedly true that psychiatry provided the intellectual and administrative leadership (not without considerable challenge even at the time), it can still be maintained that the field of child guidance and the form of child guidance clinics as agencies developed largely in response to the needs of the field of social work.

Training was one of the prime objectives of the Commonwealth Fund program. Even though the institutions were directed by psychiatrists, training concentrated on the field of social work. The Bureau of Children's Guidance, established in 1921, was an arm of the New York School of Social Work and had almost no role in the training of psychiatrists and psychologists. Its successor, the Institute for Child Guidance, was in existence from 1927 to 1933; while only 32 psychiatrists and 15 psychologists completed a year's training, fully 174 social work students were educated during these years. Another 115 social work students were trained in the institute for periods ranging from one quarter to three quarters of a school year (Lowrey & Smith, 1933).

The two training institutions established under Commonwealth Fund auspices, the Bureau of Children's Guidance (1921) and the Institute for Child Guidance (1927), still looked for cooperation from outside agencies, but both made early decisions to accept for treatment only those cases "in which the Bureau could carry the full responsibility for treatment and where there seemed to be at least potential cooperation from strategic persons in the environments of the children" (Lee & Kenworthy, 1929, p. 269). The focus was upon the work of the child guidance clinic and only secondarily upon the help which could be obtained from others who also had responsibility for the child.

The Commonwealth Fund demonstration clinics, which accepted social work trainees from their inception, also tended to emphasize a training function in the clinical setting. A not insignificant consideration in the staffing and supervisory arrangements of these early clinics was the presence of social work trainees on the staff. The demonstration clinics in St. Louis, Norfolk, Los Angeles, and Philadelphia all had social work trainees from the beginning. Moreover, the training needs of the institutions exerted strong pressure upon the selection of cases and upon the definition of a "good case" and "adequate treatment." The idealized training situation, developed so that trainees could see what was considered "best" in child guidance work, may have contributed toward the development of distinct constraints in the populations and the problems with which most later clinics worked (Stevenson & Smith, 1934; Stevenson, personal communication).

The choice to work with the individual, in contrast to an attempt to work with the larger social structure, is puzzling. In light of the virtual impossibility of meeting the immense demand for service by techniques of individual treatment, the decision to concentrate on individual cases calls for an explanation. That social workers eagerly embraced the doctrines and methods of psychoanalysis is only partly explained by the power of psychoanalytic concepts. The problems with which the field of social work was struggling might as easily have led to the development of an applied sociology. For some light on the issue of why social work took a particular direction, we shall briefly examine the history of the professional development of the social work field.

professionalization in social work

By 1899, there were two strong rival modes of operation in social work. One of these was the settlement house movement, devoted to community organization and the use of political and governmental power to gain constructive social change. (See Chapter 5.)

The second was the charity organization society, which grew out of the custom of private alms. As private philanthropy grew, intensive methods of investigation were developed to ensure that an unworthy recipient of charity did not dupe the donor and waste the largesse. Gradually the leaders recognized the need to provide a broader helping service, because the workers were able to conceptualize the problem of poverty as more than a lack of money. What began as casework to determine eligibility for charity became a method of diagnosis of the social and interpersonal needs of the family as a prelude to effective treatment. The workers of the charity organization societies generally were not concerned with the social and economic bases of poverty. Criticism would have been quite surprising for the charity societies were in part designed to show that their wealthy founders did have humanitarian concerns. The casework at first was carried out largely by untrained volunteers, but little by little the philanthropic agencies began to organize training programs both for volunteers and for the increasing number of full-time, paid workers. Experiments with summer institutes soon led to the development of full-time social work schools; by 1919 there were 17 such schools in the country (Cohen, 1958; Pumphrey & Pumphrey, 1961). While the ostensible need was to produce more effective and more efficient workers, the seeds of professionalism were being sown.

At this period, when women at all levels were entering the business and industrial world, the best educated sought new opportunities (Klein, 1946; Smuts, 1959; Flexner, 1966). The early volunteer social workers were predominantly upper-class women while the pioneers in professional social work were frequently both upper-class and college-educated. They sought significance in their lives by engaging in humanitarian and charitable activites (Addams, 1910). The meaning of these activities was enhanced by national and international recognition accorded to Jane Addams, Edith and Grace Abbott, Julia Lathrop, Florence Kelley, Lillian Wald, and many others in the field.

Viola Klein (1946) has stated that women and others having minority-group status tend to flow into new professions rather than into established ones. The barriers of tradition surely loomed higher in law, medicine, and the clergy than in the new field of social work. Among the women entering the social work field there was a conscious desire for professional status (Jarrett, 1918; Southard & Jarrett, 1922). That desire continues as an issue in social work, as is made clear in Cohen's (1958) discussion.

As social work gained in prestige and as the field grew, it began drawing women from a broader segment of society. As we have noted, the earlier workers were upper-class volunteers, pioneers, and even "fiery radicals," as Southard and Jarrett (1922) state. The first group of settlement house workers and visiting teachers were predominantly from Wellesley, Vassar, Smith, Radcliffe, and similar institutions. The first group of 70 psychiatric social workers were largely recruited from the women's colleges which, then as now, served the upper classes. The later workers, no longer of the same background,[6] came seeking economic advantage and upward social mobility (Davis, 1959). This change in background, motivation, and training of the psychiatric social worker in particular presents a set of variables demanding close attention, for the social worker is not only the gatekeeper in the child guidance clinic, but provides most of the day-to-day service.

It was in this context of a strong movement toward professional status that Abraham Flexner, a prime mover in the reform of medical education, addressed the National Conference of Charities and Corrections in 1915 on the question of whether or not social work was a profession. He stated six criteria for a profession: "professions involve essentially intellectual operations with large individual responsibility; they derive their raw material from science and learning; this material they work up to a practical and definite end; they possess an educationally communicable technique; they tend to self-organization; they are becoming increasingly altruistic in motivation . . ." (Flexner, 1961, p. 303). Flexner concluded that social work met the criteria of intellectuality and of altruism, but he questioned the degree of independent responsibility the social worker exercised. He also questioned the specificity of the aims of the field, particularly as the divergent settings and goals influenced the ability to communicate a definite body of knowledge and technique.

Flexner's careful statement came as a strong challenge to the developing field, leading many to seek a definable approach which would enable social work to qualify as a profession. It was not long after Flexner's address that Mary Richmond (1917) published her classic work, *Social Diagnosis*. With this text on social casework methodology, Mary Richmond intended to formalize a communicable body of technique, applicable to the diverse settings in which social workers were found. Her intent is clearly stated in the preface to an extraordinarily comprehensive work:

> . . . in essentials, the methods and aims of social case work were or should be the same in every type of service, whether

---

[6] White (1953) has shown that in the recent past, social work ranks higher in prestige among students of lower-class backgrounds than among those from the middle and upper classes.

the subject was a homeless paralytic, the neglected boy of drunken parents, or the widowed mother of small children. . . . The division of social work into departments and specialties was both a convenience and a necessity; fundamental resemblances remained, however. . . . It seemed to me then, and it is still my opinion that the elements of social diagnosis, if formulated, should constitute part of the ground which all social caseworkers could occupy in common, and that it should become possible in time to take for granted, in every social practitioner, knowledge and mastery of those elements, and of the modifications in them which each decade of practice would surely bring (Richmond, 1917, p. 5).

The availability of a work as complete and as thorough as *Social Diagnosis* was one important influence leading toward an emphasis on casework with the individual.[7] However, still another important influence came from the acceptance of psychoanalytic thinking by educated people in the United States. As Cohen puts it, ". . . the search for a method occurred just at the time the impact of psychoanalysis was being felt. Did social work, in its haste for professional status, reach out for a ready-made methodology for treating sick people, thus closing itself off from the influence of developments in the other social sciences?" (Cohen, 1958, pp. 120–121).

The First World War provided still another strong impetus toward the development of methodology directed to treatment of the individual. The war had produced a large number of neuropsychiatric casualties. To care for the shell-shocked veterans, a division of neuropsychiatry was developed within the army. In July of 1918, Smith College, with the cooperation of the Boston Psychopathic Hospital, announced a training program for psychiatric social workers to assist in the rehabilitation of the mentally and emotionally disturbed. E. E. Southard (1918), then chief psychiatrist at Boston Psychopathic, and Mary C. Jarrett, (1918), then chief social worker at the Boston Psychopathic,

---

[7] The importance placed on Richmond's book may be assessed from the following statement by Additon criticizing casework with girls in Philadelphia: "Clearly such evidence as is usually assembled is inadequate as a basis for diagnosis; yet, since 1917, when *Social Diagnosis* was published, social workers have had before them clear and positive statements as to the necessity of a diagnostic summary (Additon, 1928, p. 107).

were key figures in the development of the new program.[8] Intensive courses were given over an eight-week summer period, and students were sent to field placements in Boston, New York, Philadelphia, and Baltimore for six months. The following year, in keeping with their plans, Smith College expanded the course into a permanent school under the name of the Smith College Training School for Social Work.

> The purpose in view was to educate women[9] so that they might help in getting up the social history of cases presented for diagnosis to psychiatrists, that they might be of use in the treatment of such cases, and that finally they might serve in the social readjustment of psychopathic cases discharged from hospitals. The interest of the moment was of course in mental and nervous disorders resulting from the war, but they were assured that this class of disorders was by no means confined to war conditions and that the profession for which they proposed to train would be a permanent one (Neilson, 1919, pp. 59–60).

As we have indicated earlier, the trend toward work with the individual was accelerated by the fact that the alternative movement in social work, the settlement house, was declining in influence and prestige. Had they spoken out about the inadequacy of an individual, treatment-oriented approach in professional training, the settlement house workers probably would not have been heard.

The needs of the social work profession for the development of a professional methodology; the availability of the professional method of casework; the increasing popularity of psychoanalytic thinking, to

[8] A brief history of the antecedents of psychiatric social work and a good view of what practice was like in that field in its earliest years may be found in Southard and Jarrett's classic work, *The Kingdom of Evils* (1922). A detailed history of the growth of psychiatric social work is provided by French (1940).

[9] There are several determinants of the almost exclusive selection of women for the first program in psychiatric social work. One was the First World War. Because men were the shell-shocked veterans, the Smith College program was conceived as a contribution by a women's group toward the war effort. Another may be gleaned from a statement by Cook, who asserted that Dr. Southard felt that "women passed through more changes of an emotional sort in one year than men do in five, and yet are more rational than men" (Cook, 1953, quoted in Cohen, 1958, p. 133). A third is found in Viola Klein's (1946) assertion that marginal people, women, and minority group members tend to flow into new professions rather than into the established ones. The domination of the field by women in its beginnings gave it a direction which only recently has begun to show signs of change.

which psychiatric social workers were exposed from the very beginning;[10] the need to work with World War I veterans; and the ultraconservative political climate of the early 1920's led social work to develop a focus on the individual. It took but a decade for the child guidance clinic to become an agency oriented entirely toward intramural, intra-psychic therapies, and entirely away from goals of social reform, or even institutional change.

professionalization and the process of change

Originally, the child guidance clinics were meant to serve, and did serve, a low-income population. The demonstration clinic in St. Louis received 74 percent of its caseload from the Juvenile Court, but it was

[10] Among the people who taught in the original Smith College summer session were J. J. Putnam, William Healy, H. W. Frink, and A. A. Brill, all well-known analysts. Jessie Taft, who became so identified with the Rankian viewpoint, was also an instructor in that first summer session. Others with a differing orientation such as E. E. Southard, Lawson Lowrey, and Adolph Meyer taught at that first session (Spaulding, 1918).

George S. Stevenson, who was a resident at the Phipps Psychiatric Clinic of Johns Hopkins in 1918, recalls that some of the first psychiatric social work students were sent there for field experience. The girls sat on the steps of the clinic in the evening and sang their college songs, many of which were Freudian parodies. We are indebted to Dr. Stevenson, whose prodigious memory retained the two following ditties. The first was sung to the tune of "I'm wild, simply wild over Harry."

> I'm wild, simply wild over Freud,
> With his psychoanalysis, we're overjoyed.
> Our libido knows no fright,
> We dissect our dreams each night,
> Upon repression, transference, we delight.
> No dismay we display over sex,
> It is we who are free from complex.
> But we know from what we dream,
> That you are not what you seem,
> We are hep full of pep over Freud.

The second song was a parody on "There's a long, long trail a-winding, into the land of my dreams."

> There's a wrong, wrong trend that's trying
> To get you way off the track
> But until you're psychoanalyzed, you never will get back.

soon realized that children seen in the Juvenile Court[11] had long been known to schools and to other social agencies. It became clear that the clinics would be better off serving other settings such as the schools and social agencies if the work of prevention were to be carried on more effectively, and so the referral sources increased.

The Dallas demonstration clinic received referrals from the courts, social agencies, and schools, as well as from private physicians and parents. The full figures are not readily available, but in Dallas perhaps 30 percent of the cases were referred from sources likely to serve middle- or upper-income populations. In the Twin Cities clinic some 25 percent of the cases were essentially self-referred. Similarly, in Cleveland, 24 percent and in Philadelphia 33 percent were referred by parents or relatives (Stevenson & Smith, 1933). Healy and Bronner (1948) point out the same pattern held true for the Judge Baker clinic. By 1948, 60 percent of the cases were family referred.

Parents' requests for help at first were viewed as troublesome because the staff of the child guidance clinic would have to carry the entire burden of evaluation and treatment. The clinics wanted to maintain the contact with the various social agencies and the schools precisely because the contacts were a means of educating the workers from those agencies, in accordance with the original purposes of the clinics. Moreover, self-referred cases were expensive to handle because the clinic had to do all of the work of taking histories and social investigation. However, it also became apparent that seeing self-referred cases was a way of carrying the work of child guidance into other segments of the population, and finally these cases were accepted as a means of reaching the middle classes (Stevenson, personal communication).

In order to appreciate the way in which clinic practices and samples have changed, one can refer to Furman (1965) and Furman, Sweat, and Crocetti (1965). Public clinics supported exclusively by

----

[11] E. K. Wickman (personal communication), psychologist with the early clinics, has suggested that the opportunities for treatment provided by the Juvenile Court were very poor, and this too led to dissatisfaction with the affiliation with the court. All that could be accomplished in many instances was an evaluation which may or may not have had any influence on the subsequent disposition of the case. Healy and Bronner (1948) make the same point in discussing the reasons for their move from Chicago to Boston. Stevenson (personal communication) also feels the broadening of objectives from preventing delinquency to dealing with mental hygiene problems generally was in part a consequence of the frustration of trying to work with the court in St. Louis.

funds from a government subdivision serve low-income populations, while the clinics operating under voluntary auspices, the progeny of the demonstration clinics, serve upper-income populations. Self-referred cases constitute less than 3 percent of the load of publicly supported clinics, while more than half of the cases seen in the voluntary clinics are essentially self-referred. Similarly, in an informal survey of the population of four inner-city elementary schools, Sarason, et al. (1966) found but a handful of cases who had either been treated or even seen by the voluntary child guidance clinics of the area. They report a case in which a teacher attempted to arrange for evaluation and treatment for an inner-city child. The mother could not promise to accompany the child in the clinic visits. The clinic refused to consider the referral at all, effectively closing off that avenue of help.

When social workers influenced by psychoanalytic theory began to deal with self-referred parents, they discovered that in some cases advice to the mother about handling the child was not helpful. They found it necessary to study the parent-child relationship more carefully, and as they did, they discovered that some parents wanted and needed help for themselves (Allen, 1948). In a rather short period of time, it became a requirement that parents participate in the clinic's work if their children were to be accepted for service (Stevenson & Smith, 1933; Witmer, 1940). In fact, an early survey by Helen Witmer and her students (Witmer, 1933) showed that in many settings, child guidance was rapidly becoming therapy for mothers. The social work literature of the late 1920's and early 1930's focused on issues of therapy (French, 1940). This striking change took place despite clear evidence in the work of the visiting teachers, for example, and in the early work of the clinics themselves that many children could be helped by indirect modes of treatment, by active intervention in their situations, and by active, albeit patient, pursuit of their parents. It is true that studies by Witmer (1940) and her students (1933) showed that cases in which the parents did not cooperate were more difficult to treat or to retain in treatment, but there is no suggestion in Witmer's work that clinics attempted to deal with such parental resistance by a variation in their approach.

With this new requirement, the complexion of services provided by the guidance clinics changed, and the clientele also changed. Why was the requirement instituted?

In the 1920's, social workers needed a professional method, and the method they were taught was heavily influenced by psychoanalytic and psychiatric thinking. It is understandable that social workers came to depend on casework methods almost exclusively when we recall that the attainment of professional status was partially dependent on the conception that there was a professional casework technique.

In the 1920's, when people were inundated by popular Freud, it is a reasonable assumption that in contrast to parents who had to be pursued, the literate, articulate parent who brought the child to the clinic was likely to speak the social worker's language. Not only had that parent been exposed to the language in a narrow sense, but he was also likely to be from a background similar to the social worker's, and likely to share other aspects of the social worker's life style and values. It is not a great extrapolation, in light of present-day thinking, to infer that the client who came sharing the social worker's assumptions would be seen as a more desirable client, and may in fact have responded better to the techniques used by the social worker.

It is also a reasonable hypothesis that in the attempt to enhance the professional status of social work, the workers would have found gratification in serving a more prestigious social class.[12] E. S. Rademacher (personal communication), one of the psychiatrists with the Cleveland child guidance clinic of the 1920's, pointed out that during the late 1920's in an effort to erase the stigma associated with psychiatry and mental hygiene, clinic board members made it a practice to have their own children examined and treated.[13]

---

[12] Wilensky and Lebeaux (1958) hold a similar hypothesis concerning contemporary developments in the social work profession. In the psychiatric field, Hollingshead and Redlich (1958) reported that their analytic-psychological group (A-P) of psychiatrists who tended to treat upper-class patients were themselves upwardly mobile to a greater extent than the Directive-Organic (D-O) group who treated more of the lower-class patients. The D-O group more often came from upper-class backgrounds. Walsh and Elling (1968) report that upwardly mobile health workers had less favorable attitudes toward working with the poor than did less striving workers. Caplow (1954) concludes that occupational prestige is dependent upon the social position of the persons controlled by workers in an occupation.

[13] Viteles (personal communication) noted a similar phenomenon in Witmer's clinic. At first referrals were from schools and social agencies, but later many University of Pennsylvania alumni who had heard of the clinic brought their own children for help. It is interesting that over the years Witmer's interests shifted from retardation to, in the 1920's, the problems of the high I.Q. child. Terman's work with high I.Q. children was just beginning, and perhaps the bright child was "in the air."

For some people, it was a mark of modernity, and even a status symbol, to have a child in psychiatric treatment. The early use of the clinics by upper-class members of society was to influence what was considered a desirable patient by clinic workers. The derivation of prestige from an occupation serving a more prestigious clientele may well have been a consideration for an upwardly mobile group seeking professional status, in contrast to the considerations attracting the early settlement house workers or the early charity organization society volunteers.

Obviously, the hypotheses and the historical reconstruction we have advanced must be taken as tentative because the evidence necessary to support the picture is not readily available. However, we have suggested that the details of practice, the methods used, and the populations served are determined in no small part by the broader social and cultural forces which exert subtle effects upon the operations of the mental health professional. While we like to think as mental health professionals that our procedures are largely determined by objective, empirical considerations, these hypotheses suggest that the mental health professional necessarily has to broaden his theoretical perspective if he is to understand his own practices. Obviously empirical verification is difficult, but certain of the elements can be tested. For example, it would be most instructive to conduct a study of the change in social class and ethnic backgrounds of psychiatric social workers over the years. Similarly, a study of the concomitant changes in social class, racial, ethnic, and educational backgrounds of the users of clinic facilities would probably provide some meaningful evidence. Helen Witmer's (1933) survey has shown that at one point treatment in child guidance clinics was largely treatment of parents by social workers, a factor consistent with the increasing focus on the individual case and the increasing need on the part of the social workers to apply the professional techniques they had acquired.

The child guidance clinic was initially intended to treat social problems indigenous to lower-class populations. As time went on the clinic changed, and as it changed, so did the clientele it served. Viewed in the broader context of the social and intellectual forces shaping the development of social work, the later focus on techniques of individual treatment, in contrast to efforts to manipulate the gross social environment, becomes much more comprehensible.

the fate of cooperative treatment

One basic concept underlying the demonstration clinics was that of indirect service and cooperative treatment. The clinics were to evaluate a child, and then on the basis of that evaluation, they were to recommend treatment. The therapy was to be carried out by someone else, frequently under continued supervision and guidance from the clinic. Such a service pattern was desirable not only for its economic feasibility, but it was viewed as a therapeutically preferable mode of functioning. The clinic helped workers in other community agencies to become more effective in handling mental health problems in their own settings, reducing the need for outside services.

This pattern of service dropped out for the most part within a relatively few years. By the 1930's, such an emphasis in clinic practice was probably much more the exception than the rule, although clinics continued to maintain various consultative services (Schumacher, 1948). The Institute for Child Guidance (Lowrey & Smith, 1934) maintained a "one day" consultation service with other agencies, for example, but its basic interest was in treating children and their parents directly.

The change in practice brought a change in the type of problems the clinics handled. Stevenson and Smith (1933) and Witmer (1940) point out that for both the voluntary and state-supported clinics a rough sequence of referrals occurred. First the clinics were sent those who were gross mental defectives, those who had a variety of neurological disabilities, and delinquents who had been untouched by any other mode of help. A little later the schools sent aggressive, disruptive children. Finally, frequently in response to the clinics' program of educating referral sources, children were referred who were shy, withdrawn, who had habit disorders, or some other relatively circumscribed psychological problem.

There are a number of reasons for this change in population. Some relate to the training needs of the developing mental health professions, particularly social work. To some unknown degree, in many of the early clinics, and explicitly in the training centers, the Bureau for Children's Guidance and the Institute for Child Guidance, cases were accepted for treatment because of their teaching potential. The Bureau and the Institute both indicated that they consciously attempted to maintain a caseload appropriate for teaching purposes and that they consciously intended to develop within their own walls an atmosphere in which training, research, and teaching could be carried out without any pressure to service the community. Both Bureau and Institute indicated that they did not believe their intake policies seriously limited the kinds of cases which came to them. However, one cannot help but believe that students who were trained in such settings must have come away with definite conceptions about what made for a treatable case.

The basis on which cases were selected in the Bureau was not made explicit. Since an important mode of teaching was casework evaluation from the point of view of the "ego-libido" method, one can guess that cases useful in demonstrating the principles would be selected, if not for treatment, then for presentation for teaching purposes (Lee & Kenworthy, 1929). The Institute for Child Guidance, coming a few years later, was also explicit in desiring to select cases for treatment, and since the staff of the Institute was involved in innovating treatment methods with both children and parents, one may also guess that to some degree selection of cases was dependent upon the interests of clinical instructors and research teams at that time. Lowrey and Smith (1934), in their discussion of the Institute of Child Guidance, point out that the Institute's inception coincided with a growing interest in the field at large in psychotherapeutic methods. The cases which were selected were those likely to fit the demands of individual therapy. By the 1930's, the "ticket of admission" to a child guidance clinic was a complaint that the child was "nervous" (Milton Senn, personal communication).

Training considerations were also a reason for dropping the practice of cooperative treatment in the Institute. "Cooperative service was attempted in the earlier years, but abandoned because it did not fit into the training program; when social treatment was carried by the referring agency and psychiatric service by the Institute—the usual division of responsibility in this type of service—the training caseload was thrown out of balance" (Lowrey & Smith, 1934, p. 8). Note the assumption that it was not sufficiently valuable to teach young psychiatrists to work on a cooperative basis with outside agency workers. It is nowhere clear that the service was abandoned because it was found insufficiently beneficial to patients, or because it was unfeasible, although success of treatment did depend on the calibre of workers in the cooperating agency.

The clinic staffs came to feel they were most helpful with children whose difficulties were of relatively recent origin or of lesser severity, and so they tended to concentrate on those kinds of problems. What is most paradoxical about this situation is that the mental health professional, who started out by intending to help the community care for its mental health problem, ended with the "easiest" cases, and left the community agencies, presumably staffed with less well-trained people, with the more difficult problems.

Many of the early clinics did continue cooperative relationships with various agencies and schools, as did most of the demonstration clinics in the beginning. In many of these clinics the open case conference, which social workers from other agencies, physicians, teachers, and principals attended, was an important educational tool. These outsiders participated in the discussion and in planning the treatment, but while successful in some future instances, the open conference proved to be a mixed blessing.

Participants in these conferences suggested that several problems arose. For one, the various agency representatives were jealous of their prerogatives and defensive of their agencies. The agencies would sometimes fight about who had jurisdiction in a case, or the conferences would turn into a defense of a given agency's practice. For another, the cases which were selected for conferences frequently would be those which had more spectacular features, with the mental health professional attempting to dazzle the other participants. The psychiatrist frequently had difficulty in communicating because he was trained to talk in the abstractions of his profession and he found that others took his abstractions literally. As Wickman and others observed, mental health personnel tended to be rather naive, because the field was poorly developed. Rademacher, for example, described how a psychiatrist would diagnose a child who was unresponsive in interview as "schizophrenic" because the child was showing "flattened effect." The psychiatrists came into the area without much knowledge themselves and often without any special experience with children. They felt forced to use an inadequate and inappropriate nomenclature because they had no other.

Both Rademacher and Wickman felt that the social workers frequently made the most important contributions to case studies. The factual and detailed histories proved very helpful in understanding given cases. In fact, it is probably fair to say that psychiatry was as much influenced by social work as the other way around. The biologically oriented medical psychiatrist with little or no experience with children learned a great deal. It is likely that subsequent developments in the field of child psychiatry were shaped by the early contact with social workers (Stevenson, 1944; Rademacher, Stevenson, Wickman, personal communications).

Cooperative treatment and consultative relationships with agencies and schools ran afoul of still another problem. Schools of social work were offering training in clinical methods and in psychotherapy under the title of casework or social treatment. Although there were fervent denials that they were designed to produce "junior psychiatrists," as far as one can determine, the negations contained an important truth. In citing the apocryphal case of a young social worker who applied for a license to practice psychiatry from the New York Board of Regents, Glueck (1919) was doing more than giving voice to the attitude of "professional preciousness" (Sarason, et al., 1966) detectable in the medical profession from the earliest days of psychiatric social work.[14] Glueck, associated with the New York School of Social Work since 1917 and medical director of the Bureau of Children's Guidance, was developing the more salient point that the psychiatry of the day was a medical psychiatry, not really adapted to the needs of the agency worker.

It appears that little thought was given to integrating psychiatric teaching with the work of the setting which was to use it. While consciously disclaiming the intent to do so, psychiatrists apparently tried to teach social workers and others to think and to act as psychiatrists. In some instances, social workers were even taught to do neurological tests such as the knee-jerk reflex (Stevenson, personal communication).

An example is found in Levy's (1952) discussion of the temporal course of the consultative relationship between social agencies and psychiatrists. The Kraeplinian psychiatry of the day focused on diagnosis and many of the psychiatrists trained in mental hospitals knew nothing else. In their relationships with other groups, the psychia-

---

[14] Some of those who discussed Southard's (1914) paper describing the functioning of the psychopathic hospital express such concerns very clearly. See Southard and Jarrett (1922) for additional evidence of "professional preciousness." It might also be noted here that the American Orthopsychiatric Association in 1923 came about as a separate professional group in part at least because of the opposition within the American Psychiatric Association to the child psychiatrist-social worker relationship (Levy, 1952; Levy, personal communication; Stevenson, personal communication).

trists first provided them with the labels of psychopathology. As Levy (1952) indicates, it seemed to reassure agency personnel to know they were dealing with a mentally deficient youngster or with an ambulatory schizophrenic, but after a while the agency personnel, having become adept at making their own diagnoses, would then ask for specific help in managing the patient in the community. At that point psychiatric knowledge proved insufficient in providing specific working recommendations and the agency personnel responsible for treatment became somewhat disenchanted. Jarrett (1920), as a social worker receiving help from the consulting psychiatrist, expresses this complaint very well. In fact, as the psychiatric education of the social worker proceeded, and as psychiatrically trained workers entered the social agencies, the need for diagnostic consultation was reduced further. Similar issues arose when psychiatrists employed the technical terminology of psychoanalysis. Either the non-psychiatric personnel learned that technical diagnoses did not readily translate into treatment programs, or they were appalled by the "down deep and dirty" interpretive concepts of an id-oriented psychoanalysis (Ridenour, 1948; Stevenson, personal communication).

It is apparent, then, that the open case conferences, consultative services, and relationships with outside agencies were not always smooth or effective. As the psychotherapeutic model took hold, it became all too easy to justify the isolation of the child guidance clinics from the surrounding community on the grounds that the demands of psychotherapy required absolute confidentiality. By the late 1930's open case conferences or cooperative treatment relationships were just about extinct. In the Philadelphia child guidance clinic, for example, there were many fewer such contacts with the community agencies than at an earlier time (Allen, 1948). By the late 1930's agencies in the community felt a distinct lack of communication with the psychiatric staff of the clinic (Senn, personal communication).

Of course, we do not mean to imply there were no effective consulting relationships. Obviously, there were many (Loring, 1920, is an example). However the problems in the relationship may have led many in agencies and in clinics to prefer to deal with their own cases, even though the leaders in the field were concerned about the isolation such an in-clinic, intra-psychic treatment orientation would produce (Lowrey, 1948). Difficulties in managing the cooperative treatment and consulting relationships and problems in relating to the social agencies led the clinics and the training centers to give up the cooperative relationships and to focus on cases they would treat themselves. Students in psychiatry and in social work were not specifically trained to handle the cooperative supervisory or consultative relationship, and in fact there is some suggestion that such training was denigrated by the students and deemphasized by the training centers. When psychoanalytic thinking came into ascendency, there was real resistance to teaching community relationships or to teaching consultation as a specific technique. The general attitude of many was that anything which was needed along such lines would be developed in the supervision of the treatment of the individual case (Lowery & Smith, 1934; Stevenson, personal communication).

In the course of time, the clinics seemed to have selected out cases amenable to the kind of treatment they wanted to offer, generally the cases offering the best prognosis for in-clinic treatment, and they left the community agencies with the more difficult problems. In this instance, as the cooperative and overlapping staffing pattern was lost, the community agencies were left without the assistance of the more highly trained mental health professional. A reflection of the totality with which the field swept toward an intra-psychic treatment orientation is the fact that *there was little or no discussion of the relationship to community agencies as a technical problem of therapeutic practice.* Although the initial intent was to change the agencies by means of the case study and the cooperative relationship, that intent was never seriously followed through.

the child guidance clinics and the schools

The demonstration clinics decided at a very early date that by the time a child came to the Juvenile Court, it was too late to prevent his delinquency. Moreover, it was apparent that many of the children seen in the court had long been known as problems to other social agencies and to the schools. The planning of the child guidance clinics included a relationship with the schools, and in fact one of the express purposes in having a psychologist on the team was the knowledge of tests[15] the psychologist could contribute to discussions with educators.[16] As the work of the clinics centered on general problems of childhood, the clinics were necessarily concerned with the schools.

The intent of the early clinics to relate closely to the schools and the importance given the work of the visiting teacher as an agent in delinquency prevention may be inferred from the Program for the Prevention of Delinquency's plan to extend the work of the visiting teacher nationally through the schools. The Bureau of Children's Guidance, as originally established, accepted referrals from five public schools only. The Commonwealth Fund and the Public Education Association maintained a visiting teacher to work in each of the five schools with which the Bureau was to be associated. The Bureau eventually extended its services to other schools both public and private (Lee & Kenworthy, 1924).[17] The Bureau had a great deal of contact with the schools. The case studies (Sayles, 1926) are replete with references to teacher comments, visits at the school with teachers, and conferences with administrators. In individual cases, good working relationships considerably enhanced treatment. The report on the Institute for Child Guidance, written about five years after the Bureau ceased to function, does not discuss relationships with the schools (Lowrey & Smith, 1933).

The demonstration clinic in Minneapolis kept in close touch with

[15] Although Healy, and Witmer before him, had made extensive use of tests, the 1920's was the decade in which mass testing became popular. Group tests of intelligence, developed during the First World War, spread rapidly. Wickman, one of the first psychologists with the demonstration clinics, received his first training in individual testing as part of the Army program to validate group tests, another effect of war on professional functioning (E. K. Wickman, personal communication). Even had the earlier clinics not used them, with the spread of intelligence tests in the 1920's, the new clinics probably would have been forced to react to public demand.

[16] In the early days, the psychologist's major therapeutic role was that of the educational tutor or remedial specialist (Stevenson & Smith, 1934).

[17] While the Bureau itself maintained close relationships with a number of schools, one does not have to read between the lines to see that the relationship with the schools was far from smooth. The Bureau started out to work with four elementary schools and one high school. In the course of time three of the four elementary schools were dropped and three new ones were added. The Bureau's report says only that "The principals of the schools concerned were interested in the program and extended cordial cooperation." By implication, there was disinterest and a lack of cooperation in some quarters. Once again it must be emphasized that the early clinics tended not to see the problem of relating to the schools as a technical concern, and the issues were not studied.

the public schools, maintaining cooperative relationships with the visiting teachers of the school system and with workers from other agencies. In Los Angeles, the demonstration clinic worked closely with the psychological clinic of the public school, which had a staff of well-trained social workers. The clinic staff also acted as consultant to the California State Board of Education in establishing requirements for school counselors, helped to develop a plan for dealing with emotionally disturbed children in three municipal school systems, and offered a summer course for teachers.

We cannot pretend to know all of the elements which led the child guidance clinics away from the schools and toward independent treatment. We have listed some of the issues above. However, we cannot help but believe that a primary factor in the eventual dissolution of relationships, even where the relationships were clinically effective, was the profound difference between mental health workers and teachers in their orientation toward child development and the behavior and emotional problems of children.

The classic research[18] in this area was E. K. Wickman's (1928) work, completed while he was engaged in various child guidance activities with the Commonwealth Fund's program. Wickman obtained measurement of the differential attitudes held by teachers toward undesirable behavior in children. He compared the weightings given by teachers to various behavior problems with those given by a sample of mental health workers. The merits and deficiencies of Wickman's research are not at issue here. A critique of his studies and a review of subsequent work may be found in Beilin (1962). Suffice it to say that Wickman was very careful to qualify his findings and he himself pointed out a major issue in his work which limits its interpretation. Mental hygienists were asked to rate the behavior problems in terms of their significance for future adjustment, while teachers' ratings were in terms of the degree of maladjustment represented by the immediate problem.

Given these limitations, Wickman found that teachers' ratings of seriousness fell into four groups, in decreasing order of seriousness.

A. Immoralities, dishonesties, transgressions against authority

---

[18] Wickman's study, the forerunner of a great deal of later research and still widely cited, was not acceptable as a Ph.D. dissertation. He was told that he could take it to a department of education, but that it was not psychology (E. K. Wickman, personal communication)!

    B. Violations of orderliness in classroom; application to
       school work
    C. Extravagant, aggressive personality and behavior traits
    D. Withdrawing, recessive personality and behavior traits

Mental hygienist ratings fell into the following four groups in
decreasing order of seriousness:

    A. Withdrawing, recessive personality and behavior traits
    B. Dishonesties, cruelty, temper tantrums, truancy
    C. Immoralities; violation of school work requirements;
       extravagant behavior traits
    D. Transgressions against authority; violations of order-
       liness in class

His discussion of the issues is still fresh and enlightening. Wickman conceptualized two basic forms of "evasion of social requirements,"
withdrawal and attack. He postulated that these two modes of response
were learned in relation to earlier social demands placed by parents
and they were elicited by the social demands of the school. The two
modes of response are discussed in relation to their significance for
the teacher:

> Our experimental results may be summed up in two state-
> ments: To the extent that any kind of behavior signifies
> attack upon the teachers and upon their professional
> endeavors does such behavior rise in their estimation as a
> serious problem. To the extent that any kind of unhealthy
> behavior is free from such attacking characteristics does it
> appear, to teachers, to be less difficult, less undesirable and
> less significant of child maladjustment (pp. 159–160).

Wickman goes on to discuss the teacher's handling of behavior
problems in terms of the emotional responses the behavior elicits in
the teacher:

> An inspection of the characteristic form of discipline em-
> ployed for children who are disobedient, dishonest, truant,
> disorderly, or who offend by sexual behavior, reveals the
> counter-attacking nature of the teachers' behavior. Punish-

ments in various forms and disguises are generally administered. In this connection it is essential to note that
punishment is not limited to blows to the body. Wounding
the child's pride, self-respect, and personal integrity may
not have the sinister appearance of corporal punishment but
it leaves its marks even more surely on the child and
relieves the tension of the adult. The counter-attack may
take the form of shaming the child, criticizing him before
the class, exacting confessions, requiring apologies, or
restrictions, impositions of tasks, negations, prohibitions,
admonitions, demotions. . . . In all these methods of discipline there is a display of the aggrieved adult whose authority or personal integrity has been violated. . . .

Punishment, to be legitimate, can only be applied when
it is intelligently chosen with a conception of the causes of
the behavior problem clearly in mind. Intelligent punishment
is precluded so long as behavior problems are evaluated in
relation to their frustrating character. The requirement that
the child must obey simply because "I say so" or because
the school demands it, cannot be defended rationally. That
implicit conformity to adult standards of morality, honesty,
and obedience is for the good of the child is often made
the justification for the methods of discipline that are
employed.

Insofar as the withdrawing types of behavior problems
are evaluated as of least importance, we may assume that
the teachers' behavior responses to these problems are
characterized by tolerance and indulgence. . . . The show
of dependency that is characteristic of withdrawing behavior makes for ease in classroom administration. It is
looked upon with favor. Unsocial children often attract the
favor of the teacher by applying themselves diligently to
school tasks in which they find a refuge from the difficulties
of social adjustment (pp. 162–163).

It was Wickman's view that the counterattack results only in a
fixation of the behavior, either through emphasizing the "bad self"
or through reinforcing a child's antagonism to authority. Similarly the
support that conforming behavior received in the school setting re-

inforced sick behavior. From the point of view of the mental hygienist of that day, Wickman points out that in both instances the response to a child's behavior is not dictated by an understanding of causes, but rather by the surface manifestations of behavior and the feeling the behavior calls forth in the teacher. In neither instance is the teacher's behavior rational.

While Wickman recognized the fundamental educational purpose of the school, both intellectual and social, he propounded the viewpoint that the basic problem lay not in the teacher's function, but in a lack of appreciation of the significance of the overt behavior pattern. If attacking behavior is disruptive, blind punishment is no answer. Moreover much of what was characterized as attacking behavior represented normal activities of childhood. Investigatory, experimental activity and curiosity about one's self and the world, including one's self as a sexual being, is a normal part of childhood, not to be censured but to be accepted and respected as a part of development. In addition, Wickman pointed out that the attacking child in school did not necessarily fail in life, while the "good" child of the withdrawing type was sometimes unsuccessful after leaving school.

Wickman argued that the mental health worker had a superior, i.e., more scientific view of child development, and moreover that the educator's approach was not necessarily in the child's best interests, from the point of view of the mental health worker concerned with future adaptation to the world.

Allen's (1929) paper is a sensitive appreciation of the difference in viewpoint between psychiatric social worker and teacher, particularly in relation to the teacher's exercise of authority. Allen also emphasized the problems which arise because the teacher has responsibility for a large group and the mental health worker tends to think in terms of the individual case, but her basic point is the same as Wickman's. When the teacher can attain an attitude of objectivity toward individual children and not blame herself or respond on the basis of her anger and frustration, then the teacher can act rationally to help the problem.

Since the mental health worker, however much he sympathized with the teacher's position, approached the school from the viewpoint that the teacher must change,[19] it would appear almost inevitable that

---

[19] Most of the literature has been written by mental health workers. It would be most instructive to have more data from the educator's viewpoint. We do not know in what ways it would be desirable for the mental health worker to change in concepts and approach if he is to relate meaningfully to educators.

conflict would develop. Wickman implies as much when he says that change in attitudes is not readily accomplished in adults. It is our guess that the differences in viewpoint between teacher and mental health worker, a difference which seems to crop up even today (Grant & Stringer, 1964; Sarason, et al., 1966; Newman, 1967), must have contributed to the gulf between them. Although there is no direct evidence at this point to show how the child guidance clinics retreated from extensive contact with schools, it is our guess that the retreat occurred because the mental health professional did not take the problem of relating to the schools as a serious technical issue worthy of intensive study.

While not immediately germane to the chief argument we are developing here, Wickman's prescriptions for improvement in the school situation are worthy of mention. They reflect the mental hygienist's viewpoint of forty years ago, but they clearly have relevance for today's teachers. Wickman recommended that teachers get improved knowledge of normal child behavior, including intellectual, social, and sexual development. He recommended that teachers receive training in diagnosing and treating children's behavioral problems by learning to think in terms of causes and by learning to direct action toward the emotional and experiential factors producing the problems. He further recommended that some way should be developed to help teachers withstand the shock of having to deal with the raw impulses of childhood so that the teachers themselves would gain better control of their own emotional states.

It would appear that a "geopolitical goal" of the mental health worker, if he is to develop a truly preventive approach, is to enter fully into the training of teachers. To this day, that goal has been reached only in the most sporadic way by the mental health field. We surmise that the mental health worker will not be able to develop fully satisfactory relationships with the school system until he does become fully involved in the training of teachers and administrators.

a case study

In order to provide some appreciation of the nature of treatment in the early child guidance clinic, the following case material is presented. Much of what follows is extracted from Sayles' (1926) little volume of case reports from the Bureau of Children's Guidance. The cases, designed to show in detail how the clinics worked, were intended for an audience of agency social workers, teachers, probation officers, public health nurses, and parents rather than for psychiatrists and psychiatric social workers. In the following material, taken from one case, we shall emphasize the various therapeutic activities undertaken on behalf of the child. We shall also emphasize the contacts the workers made with the home, the school, and other agencies. The reader familiar with present-day child guidance clinic practices might be interested in asking himself how such activities would be considered by a staff exclusively oriented toward psychotherapy.

Mildred Martin was brought to the clinic at age twelve, so unable to do school work that she had been placed in a first-grade class upon transferring from a parochial to a public school. "Apathetic, unsocial, sullen, she seemed to have retired into an inner world of her own to such a degree that those who observed her had become seriously alarmed about her mental state" (p. 7). The visiting teacher who brought Mildred to the clinic[20] had visited the child's home to discover that Mildred's mother was devoted, sober, and industrious, but that her father was an alcoholic and that Mildred had been under treatment for congenital syphilis. It was the visiting teacher assigned to the school who took the child's history from the mother in her own home. We shall omit details of the family and their history, for these are unimportant for our present purposes. The very thorough history obtained by the visiting teacher was sufficient for the clinic's purposes. No further visits from the mother to the clinic were required.

Mildred was supposed to report to a medical clinic once a week for her syphilis shots. The visiting teacher discovered she was a difficult patient, often screaming, kicking, and biting the doctors and nurses, slipping out of the clinic before her shots, and pretending to her mother that she had them. The visiting teacher treated this aspect of her problem by giving Mildred a note to the medical clinic social worker who would send back a reply.[21] This method of checking up on her progress improved both her attendance and her behavior at the clinic.

[20] The clinic procedure did not require that the parent bring the child for help. The social worker was very willing to make a home visit and to obtain the necessary information from the mother in her own home. Such a practice would be unusual in most clinics today.

[21] The social worker did not hesitate to enter into various aspects of the child's life. The contacts were not restricted to clinic visits.

The girl was seen by a psychologist, who found her unresponsive but cooperative, and he obtained an I.Q. of 97. The woman psychiatrist who saw Mildred *did the physical examination herself.*[22] The child was more responsive with the psychiatrist, and produced enough to permit the psychiatrist to conclude she was probably not in an early stage of dementia praecox, but rather that she had a deep emotional difficulty related to the problems uncovered in the school and home environments. Mildred was taken into therapy and while not resistant to coming, she did express some unhappiness about having to come to the clinic because she was escorted there by the visiting teacher.

Following the series of examinations and the completion of the history by the visiting teacher, the clinic staff worked out a plan of treatment. One of the first elements in the plan involved permission for the child to arrive for her clinic appointments unescorted by the visiting teacher. The visiting teacher went to her home and worked out the arrangement with her mother. She asked the mother to change Mildred's room because Mildred had been fighting with a sister who teased her a great deal.

The social worker (it is not clear whether this is the visiting teacher or the clinic worker) continued to visit the girl's home and to work with the mother. The nature of the contact may be seen from the social worker's notes:

> Explained to Mrs. Martin how very sensitive Mildred is about her school work and urged that she use every means possible to keep her sisters from taunting her about it or from comparing her progress with that of her younger sister. Suggested that they all treat Mildred just as they would any other child her age, emphasizing the fact that now she is having the better school opportunities she will learn very rapidly and will soon be in her own class. Told her that if the family encouraged her and expected her to

---

[22] Healy instituted the practice of the psychiatrist doing physicals in child guidance work. Later, when psychoanalytic concepts guided psychotherapeutic practices, many psychiatrists stopped doing physicals on the grounds that the physical represented either a castration threat or a sexual assault, and therefore was antitherapeutic (Senn; Stevenson, personal communication). Other considerations led clinics to minimize physicals. Allen (1948), for example, felt parents would be confused if the clinic emphasized physical exams.

succeed she would be happier and would make better progress. Pointed out the danger of sensitive people withdrawing into themselves, brooding over their disabilities and difficulties and developing a set feeling of inferiority. Suggested that if there was anything Mildred did more successfully than her sisters, this be picked out for special commendation and attention. Suggested that it is better for Mildred to talk things out than to shut herself up and withdraw (Sayles, 1926, pp. 27–28).

The notes suggest the worker was highly directive and specific in her recommendations to the mother. The worker remarked at how able the mother was in grasping and implementing suggestions. There is little to indicate that the worker found it necessary to work through with Mrs. Martin her feelings about the child or about the suggestions.[23]

The social worker had very little luck in working with Mr. Martin. She tried to visit him in his home repeatedly and wrote to him on several occasions. She even located an employment opportunity for him, but he never responded. Despite the failure to achieve any change, or for that matter much contact with Mr. Martin, the worker never expressed any sense of discouragement, nor did she seem to feel it futile to pursue her client.

Part of the treatment program called for the child to engage in a variety of activities designed to give her interests outside of herself and to take her out of her home for definite periods of time, for her home was described as a depressing influence. The social worker carried out the "social treatment": first obtaining Mrs. Martin's consent, the social worker found a Girl Scout troop, took the child to the first meeting, and continued to encourage her to attend meetings until she was well established in the troop.[24] The clinic furnished her with money for her uniform and for dues when necessary. Mildred eventually became an enthusiastic scout.

[23] Many today would say that such direction in interviews would be to no avail because the parent would distort the advice or would execute it improperly due to emotional involvement with the child. While true in many instances, it apparently is not always true, as Healy's cases also suggested.

[24] The social worker was not concerned about the mother's lack of responsibility, nor did she hesitate to pursue the plan vigorously even though the child was resistant.

During the first month of treatment, the worker also took the child on an all-day outing to a museum, to lunch, and the Hippodrome, and helped her to know the public library. Later on in their relationship, the worker learned that the girl had a fondness for sewing and knitting. She encouraged Mildred to make Christmas gifts for friends and family, taking the child to her own home for a lesson and for supper.[25] The worker obtained a place for Mildred in a seaside home for the summer as well and arranged for financial support through a relief agency which had worked with the Martin family.

From the very beginning of treatment, Mildred's visiting teacher stayed in close touch with the school situation. Tutoring had been arranged by the visiting teacher. The clinic social worker visited Mildred in her classroom and had frequent conferences with the visiting teacher who, in turn, had periodic contacts with the child. At one point, when the child, disappointed about an expected promotion, was truant, the visiting teacher went to her home to discuss the problem with her and arranged for a school supervisor to visit the child in her classroom to explain the promotion problem to her.

After one mid-year promotion, when it was discovered that the child was not doing too well, the clinic social worker, at the suggestion of the treating psychiatrist, interviewed her new teacher and discovered the child needed additional help. A tutor was suggested; the psychiatrist broached the subject with her in her next interview, only to discover that Mildred was concerned that others would see her with the tutor if it were done in the assembly where she had been tutored previously. The visiting teacher appreciated her concern and arranged for after-school tutoring, away from the public assembly room. Mildred was then able to work very successfully with her tutor.[26]

The psychotherapy program is not described in any great detail. Mildred had regular appointments with the psychiatrist, but the frequency of appointments is not indicated in the original case study, nor

---

25 Such practices would likely be frowned upon, if not actually prohibited, in many contemporary clinics. A worker who took a client to her own home would likely be accused of overidentifying or of having rescue fantasies. Part of the problem may have to do with increased "professionalism." Schoolteachers also express conflict about whether it is professionally correct to have a closer, more personal relationship with their children (Sarason, et al., 1966).

26 It is interesting that the helping personnel did not feel it was essential for Mildred to confront her "irrational" fear of being seen with a tutor.

is there much to indicate the nature of the psychiatrist's approach. It does seem that the child was seen regularly, with the initial interview lasting half an hour. The psychiatrist acted as a friend who encouraged her to express her problems and seemed to support her in various ways; the psychiatrist tried to understand her viewpoint and make life seem less desperate and hopeless to her.

Apparently the psychiatrist helped her to anticipate and to work through some of her feelings about the plans made for her. Moreover, distressing matters which were discovered in the interviews and which could be corrected in the environment were corrected following the psychiatrist's recommendations to the clinic social worker or to the visiting teacher. As the child gained confidence in the psychiatrist, she apparently used her to ventilate some of her feelings about her poor home situation. The psychiatrist did not attempt to elicit the child's feelings of hostility toward her drunken father, but on the contrary seemed to support her in her tender solicitude for the man.

Mildred progressed beautifully under the treatment, which continued over a period of about two years. A follow-up about three years after the end of treatment indicated Mildred was a happy, successful adolescent with normal heterosexual interests. The family situation had improved somewhat, although there was no important change in the father. As his children did things which enabled him to feel a sense of pride in them, he apparently responded with somewhat greater warmth and affection for the entire family, but he continued to drink heavily from time to time.

Of course, successful cases were selected for presentation in this source, but it does seem that many of the therapeutic tactics would not be employed in today's typical psychotherapeutically oriented clinic. It is certainly possible that so much manipulation of a child's life might take away from a sense of responsibility and dilute the effectiveness of a psychotherapeutic relationship. On the other hand, the results in selected cases certainly would not support the view that all such treatment was superficial, or inevitably ineffective, a view extreme proponents of psychotherapeutic methods are sometimes prone to expound in discussions of other approaches. The subsequent changes in clinic practice were due not to poor results with the methods employed but to other factors. The Bureau of Children's Guidance reported a success and partial success rate of better than 90 percent with methods such as those used with Mildred (Lee & Kenworthy, 1929).

summary

The privately supported community child guidance clinic that we know today is a mental health agency strongly influenced in its development by the experience of the Commonwealth Fund demonstration clinics. The latter were established in the 1920's as part of a program for the prevention of juvenile delinquency. The demonstration clinics, in their earliest conception, were designed primarily not to provide treatment for children showing psychological problems, but to enable a variety of other social, child welfare, and educational organizations to handle the problems of children in a more effective fashion. The orginal focus on juvenile delinquency seemed to reflect a continuation of the social reform thinking prevalent in the generation preceding World War I. After World War I, the nation became conservative. Individual responsibility was emphasized; social reform was a dead issue.

In the post-war period, there were many changes in the role of women and a considerable upheaval in prevalent sexual mores. While many personal, traditional beliefs were challenged, the post-war generation continued to believe in science as the answer to man's problems. In the human relations field science meant psychoanalysis and psychology. The growth of mass communication spread a variety of conflicting beliefs about proper child rearing practices and caused much parental uncertainty. It was in this context of changing values, changing sex roles, and uncertainty that the child guidance clinics offering scientific expertise grew.

It was apparent from the very beginning that a treatment service could never hope to meet service needs and that it would be necessary to develop techniques for educating the relevant settings to handle their own problems. Despite this, within a decade, the clinics moved in the direction of almost exclusively providing in-clinic treatment services to parents and children. Moreover, as they moved in this direction, contacts with other agencies and institutions were minimized and the population which was served changed from predominantly lower-class to predominantly middle-class.

It is argued that the shift toward individual treatment, in contrast to an applied sociology directed to social and institutional reform, reflected the intellectual and social spirit of the 1920's. That spirit was receptive to a belief in individual responsibility and refractory to the concept of broad social responsibility. It is further argued that the changing opportunities for women led many to enter social work with the hopes of achieving professional status. Considerations of training, forces leading toward professionalism, and desire for upward social mobility led to an emphasis on casework and therapeutic interviewing with individuals. There are a variety of suggestions that relationships with other social agencies and with the schools were not always fruitful or conflict-free. Instead of approaching the problem of relating to institutions and the problems of institutional change as technical issues, deserving consideration in their own right, the difficulties may have encouraged the further isolation of the clinics, which were then more interested in the problem of developing methods of direct treatment of individual children and their parents.

The aims, the organization, and the early experience of the Commonwealth Fund demonstration clinics and the changes over time reveal the broad and complex forces which combine to shape mental health practices, forces which mental health professionals generally ignore. The approach of the early clinics in terms of their treatment methods and their relationships to a broad variety of social agencies might well be reexamined in this day of concern about the adequacy of contemporary child guidance practice to meet the challenges presented by the imperative needs of our growing urban population.

11

social change and helping forms

We have argued that helping forms arise in response to urgent social need, and that the urgent social need is a product of social change. When the predominant ethos favors social change, people will be viewed as essentially good and the cause of problems seen in their living conditions. Helping forms will try to modify existing social institutions toward greater relevance for the immediate conditions of life and will try to develop new social institutions to provide for personal growth and development.

When the predominant social ethos is essentially conservative, when the way of life is considered good and the institutions viable, the causes of problems will be located in the individual's personal weaknesses and deficiencies. Since he is an inadequate being, he will be able to take advantage of existing opportunities only when he is brought up to par. The helping form will arise as a separate community facility whose purpose is to help individuals to adapt themselves to existing social conditions. Helping agencies' acceptance of such a purpose implicitly validates existing social norms. The person is therefore treated in a setting removed from the one in which his problem manifests itself. In the language of contemporary social theory, such a mental health facility is primarily an agent of deviance control (Scheff, 1966).

Thus far we have stated a simple correlation between the helping form and the general social ethos. In the very language in which we have expressed our views, we have revealed a bias toward solutions emphasizing changes in the social order. We admit to such a bias at this point in time, because we are writing not only to express a "correct" view of the past, but to direct the attention of the mental health professions toward a consideration of new forms of help. We do not intend to denigrate current forms of practice but rather to express our understanding of the contemporary social situation.

We began our study of history out of an enthusiasm for those accounts of the past which showed striking resemblances to the present. But then we asked ourselves to suppose that both the attempt to change social institutions and the attempt to change individuals stemmed from accurate perceptions of the social world at a given point in time. What followed? How could we understand the correlation in broader theoretical terms which would enable us to make predictions to the future?

Let us assert as a basic assumption that people organize their lives largely according to the ways in which they earn their livings. Most of the major social institutions, be they educational, legal, religious, recreational, or health, help to maintain that way of life. In the period under discussion in this book, the United States changed from a predominantly rural and agricultural society to a predominantly urban and industrial society. The cities and factories absorbed successive waves of peoples with foreign and rural folkways and mores but the social institutions of the newly developing cities were based upon traditions relevant to a vanishing social order. Because the way of life was changing, irrelevant social institutions were under pressure to change, for good and sufficient reasons. When institutions are obstructive and irrelevant, we speak of alienation of individuals from their society. The problem of alienation, whether or not that early Marxian term was used, preoccupied the attention of the progressives and the reformers of the pre-World War I period.

Customs, laws, beliefs, and values all change slowly. Systems arising from one way of life do not readily adapt to another and new social institutions are not readily created by a society which does not believe in interference with natural social evolution. When the socially concerned mental health workers of an earlier day argued that social institutions were causing problems in living, they were perfectly right.

A way of life had changed, but it took a long time and much struggle before social institutions changed to reduce alienation by serving people in terms of how people actually lived. In a later time, when the institutions had changed to some extent,[1] the problems people had were not seen as clearly related to the existence of faulty institutions, and new forms of help focused on helping individuals adapt to a new life style. Changes in the pre-World War I period centered on the schools, courts, social agencies, health and recreational facilities, housing and working conditions. Changes in the post-war period centered on manners and morals and on how people lived with themselves and with each other in the more stabilized urban, industrial society.

Historians and political scientists refer to historical periods as either reform or conservative. "Conservative" describes governments dominated by business interests or governments in which some tradition, or some conventional wisdom, to use Galbraith's (1958) helpful term, is supported. "Reform" describes the efforts of socially conscious citizens to achieve changes in the service of "the people," or changes in the service of a different view of the social order. Our reading of history suggests the term "acute social change" may be more descriptive than reform. When there are major political reforms, we suspect that it can be demonstrated that the rest of the major institutions of society are also under pressure to change. The introduction of the factory system and inventions which captured new sources of energy led to profound changes in a whole way of life, and not only to municipal reform.

The massive social problems of the present day show that once again we are in a period of acute social change. We are now experiencing the consequences of a fairly drastic shift in the way in which people earn a living. We have mastered new, powerful sources of energy, highly efficient and flexible materials and machinery, extraordinarily sophisticated devices for communication, and speedy devices for transportation.

It is no longer necessary to commit the largest proportion of human resources to ensure survival or even to provide luxuries. The need no longer exists for as many people to engage in economically useful work, as that term has been defined in the past (Galbraith,

---

[1] We do not intend any implication that the changes were caused exclusively or even largely by the efforts of social reformers. Surely they helped but the extent of their influence should not be overestimated.

1958; AFL-CIO, 1959; Brightbill, 1960; Theobald, 1961; Bazelon, 1962; DeGrazia, 1962; AFL-CIO, 1963; Charlesworth, 1964; Sarnoff, 1964).

Were government and the industrial complex to commit their resources to the acceleration of trends already in evidence, relatively few people could do most of the work. Unskilled and semi-skilled production and maintenance jobs are rapidly disappearing, while service positions, professional and technical employment, and supporting staffs are rising in numbers. According to Labor Secretary Willard Wirtz, of 4.3 million new jobs created in the six years prior to 1964, 63 percent were in state and local government and in non-profit organizations, while only 4.7 percent were in private, profit-making, non-war-related industries (Wirtz, 1964). Machlup (1962) shows that one-third of the labor force is employed in the knowledge industries. Clearly, the need for new workers to produce the goods we require is not very strong. Were it not for the problems of distribution of those economic goods, and a deeply ingrained moral principle that each man must work, we venture to guess that the number of employed people and the number of hours required of each employed person could be quite low.

The way people spend their lifetime today differs markedly from the way they did in the recent past. The work week is decreasing while vacations increase; the retirement age is earlier than ever. At the moment, each adult in this country has 45,000 more hours at his disposal than his counterpart of a century ago had during his lifetime. Even working hours are spent quite differently than they were a century ago. A reported survey of the activities of executives suggested they spent about 80 percent of work hours talking, while our own informal survey of the work activities of people in a variety of white collar, technical, and professional positions indicates that anywhere from 25 to 80 percent of the work week is spent in conference with two or more other people.

We do not know the actual proportion of time at work spent in communication and staff conferences, office parties, coffee and recreation breaks, extended luncheon engagements, conventions, retreats, and similar activities, but we venture to guess that the proportion of time that most people spend with some non-human objects as the major focus of attention during working hours has changed radically over the last few decades. If our speculation is correct, what does this imply for the concept of work?

In addition to a change in the amount and nature of work activity, most people are entering the work force at a much later age and the period of education is likely to be extended still further in the future. Children start their pre-school education as young as three and four. Nursery schools unquestionably will grow with great rapidity in the near future and day care centers for still younger children are also appearing. With an ever-increasing proportion of high school graduates opting for post-high school educations, two-year junior and community colleges are developing at least as rapidly as pre-schools. Graduate and professional schools are pressured to take in increasing percentages of college graduates. We feel that this trend will continue for not only does the increased education required to enter the labor force reflect the preponderance of highly technical positions in a mature, industrial civilization, but at the same time, it serves to keep people out of the labor market for long periods. In a day when "featherbedding" is a source of labor-management conflict, the latter consideration cannot be ignored.

In 1967, almost 30 percent of the population was in school full time as students, and we are counting only public and private elementary and secondary schools and colleges. If we included all those adults in industry and the armed forces who are in some form of full-time job training, retraining, or in-service training, those figures would add substantially to the percentage of the population being educated at any given moment. Since the years from three to 21 alone represent about 25 percent of the average expected life span, schooling may no longer be considered a preparation for life. In the United States at the present moment schooling must be considered a way of life, and the proportion of the population committed to that way of life will undoubtedly increase in the near future.

In short, the number of people necessary to do the work of the world, as we have known work in the past, is decreasing. Larger numbers of people are committing less of their lifetimes to work. More of those who are engaged in work are performing tasks radically different, and under radically different circumstances, than was true in even the recent past. Change in the way people earn their living creates tremendous strain on various social institutions, particularly those related to socialization, and to the maintenance of norms of conduct. The ongoing social change implies that changes in helping forms may be best directed to reevaluating the goals of socialization and the accompanying norms of behavior.

Freud argues that civilization, a condition of social order, requires a renunciation of instinctual expression and the development of internalized controls in the form of a conscience. Delays in gratification must be accepted and enforced. Moreover, Freud argues that for socialization to occur instinctual expression must be restricted and he points to the educator's repressive attitude toward most forms of libidinal expression in the young as evidence for his concept. Society's need for order with resultant renunciation of instinctual expression will always conflict with individual desire for unhampered libidinal satisfaction and thus discontent is inherent in civilization (Freud, 1930; Freud, 1938; Freud, 1959).

Let us add to Freud's argument the proposition that the degree of instinctual renunciation required is directly related to the amount of human energy required by any social group to earn its living. A society which masters some new source of physical energy or develops substitutes for human labor requires less human energy for its maintenance. An appropriate expansion in the permissible forms of libidinal expression should follow.[2] At one level, the viewpoint is highly oversimplified, and the closed-energy hydraulic model leaves much to be desired in microdetail. Still, the model is helpful when we consider the nature of helping forms or preventive forms in the predictable future.

Our contemporary economy makes it most attractive to shift our basic attitudes toward instinctual renunciation. Galbraith (1958) speaks of the creation of new consumer wants as a vital element if the present economy is to maintain full production and full employment, while Henry (1965) writes about the role of advertising both in creating wants and in promoting the irrational thinking which makes it easy to create wants. Henry argues that our way of life is increasingly geared to immediate gratification of consumer desires, with the consequence that there may be an erosion of our collective willingness to delay satisfactions. The press toward gratification as a consequence of available time and energy is supplemented, then, by a pull toward impulse expression through advertising and available credit.

Galbraith (1958) argues that attempting to satisfy ever-increasing consumer wants is neither a necessary aspect of a full economy, nor an essential emphasis in the life of individuals. If there were national goals and means of deciding personal worth other than contribution to pro-

2 Fuller development of the social implications of these principles may be found in Levine and Levine (in press).

duction or propensity to consume, we would be freer to consider other acceptable ways of being.

For the sake of argument, let us accept the assumption that work, as society has defined it in the recent past, is obsolete. One immediate implication is that our concepts of deviance must undergo radical change, for we can safely argue that at the heart of our concern about deviance is the problem of economic dependency. We concern ourselves somewhat with people who suffer inwardly or who do not develop fully, but we do not really consider people social problems until their personal difficulties interfere with their functioning in the economic world. In the case of a child, we attend to the problem if we fear that he will be unable to earn a living in the future.

The issue is most drastically confronted in relation to the mentally deficient child. While there are many social consequences for the family with a mentally deficient child, among the most central of parental concerns is the question: "Who will take care of him after we're gone if he cannot get an education and a good job?" Institutions try hard to educate mentally deficient children to minimal levels in reading, writing, and arithmetic, even though the positions appropriate to the attainable level of education are rapidly disappearing.[3] Moreover, with the advent of television and other audio-visual devices, one can keep up with the world and enjoy it without being able to read and write. Many of us, including the troops overseas, now correspond with friends using tape recorders instead of written letters. We might be able to save a great deal of time and heartbreaking effort if we supplied mentally deficient children with tape recorders and taught them the simple mechanics of using them.

Institutions for the mentally defective spend a great deal of time teaching handiwork, art, and sports with more success as a rule than standard academic subjects. Such studies, however, are introduced as peripheral aspects of programs and are not presented as the central activity. The products of such training are treated as compensatory accomplishments, as indices that mentally deficient children do have some social worth, but they are rarely exhibited as accomplishments significant in their own right. Arts and crafts are not respected as activities

---

[3] The jobs disappear in two ways. First, as our ideals of social justice encourage guarantees of minimum wage levels, unskilled jobs are not filled or are automated; and second, educational requirements for jobs continue to reflect what is essential for obtaining the jobs, not for performing the work (Clark, 1964).

in which people might engage full-time simply for sheer enjoyment. They are presented as supplements, as hobbies, as a nice way for the children to spend their time when they are relaxing from the effort to learn skills vital to earning a living. Imagine an institution trying to sell itself to a state legislature or to parents wholly as a place where mentally deficient children develop and enjoy the exercise of whatever skills and talents they have, irrespective of the economic usefulness of the activities. The institution would be driven out of existence. The pretense of training economically useful skills is necessary for there is no other rationale enabling us to provide for a variety of forms of personal development.

Attitudes toward sexual activity among the institutionalized mentally retarded present another curious problem. Much emotional effort is expended by institutional personnel in minimizing sexual expression among the inmates. Masturbation, homosexuality, and heterosexual interests are largely discouraged. Since sure methods of sterilization or contraception exist, there is no obvious reason why mentally deficient individuals should not be permitted to enjoy sexual pleasures as part of an institutionalized way of life. It is as if society believes very deeply that only those who are capable of taking care of themselves, in the conventional definition of that concept, are entitled to sexual pleasures. Sexuality, both in its pre-genital and in its genital manifestations, is denied to dependents, be they adults or children. The real-life sexual adventures of a wealthy movie queen excite our admiring attention, but the sexual indulgence of a woman living on welfare elicits our opprobrium.

Let us examine the issues of deviance and dependence from another vantage point. A predominant issue in the field of child guidance is the learning disorder, and the overriding concern of educators is the slow learner, a euphemism for the lower-class child who is two or more years behind grade level in academic achievement. If we examine the concept of a learning disorder carefully, we find that it means not an inability to learn anything, but an inability to learn the narrow set of intellectual skills schools teach. The same child who presents a learning disorder in the classroom may produce beautiful art work, dance with grace and elegance, be a competent athlete, or have a variety of interpersonal skills which make him popular among his peers. At the heart of the concern about such a child is not that he will be unable to develop himself in some direction, but that he will be unable to develop the particular skills which will make him employable. What is characterized as a learning disorder, an undesirable deviance, is really behavior eliciting the anxious prediction that the child will not be able to take care of himself when he grows up.

Another common complaint teachers voice is that the young child has a poor attention span. Examined in detail, the complaint really means that the child will not attend to the task the teacher sets before him. When the same child is engaged in a self-selected activity, running about the playground, earnestly painting a picture on an easel, or carefully examining a tiny crawling bug, no such deficiency in attention is demonstrated. If one asks the teacher why the child cannot be permitted to pursue his own interests, the teacher indicates that the mature person cannot always do what he wants; at some point the child will have to learn to subordinate his interests to those of the authorities responsible for his socialization. The child who will not readily accept the externally imposed tasks designed to prepare him for his place in the world is defined as "pathological."

The nomenclature of psychopathological disorders of childhood proposed by the Group for the Advancement of Psychiatry (1966) stresses deviation from some norm, with measures of acceptable variations around the norm unspecified. Thus a trait such as "significant precociousness or acceleration in intellectual development" is considered a form of deviance. So are behavior patterns characterized by: "shyness"; "exhibitionistic tendencies"; "passive, feminine boys or somewhat masculine girls who do not show actual inversion or perversion"; "mood swings"; chronically ebullient, active, though not ordinarily hyperactive . . . characterized by generally positive attitudes with much impatience over growing up and . . . a tendency toward overly responsible behavior of a pseudomature type"; and sociosyntonic personality disorders which include "personality pictures that derive from cultures other than that of the majority group." Moreover the description of such traits in an authoritative and semi-official diagnostic manual of psychiatric disorder implies they ought not to be, that they are symptoms of sickness, and that children with such characteristics should be treated to attain "the comfortable fit of an individual into a particular set of social circumstances" considered to be an important sign of the healthy personality.

The mental health professional functions as an agent of deviancy control and deviance is defined in terms of variation from "the comfortable fit of an individual into a particular set of social circumstances." If we look further at these concepts and ask about the "particular set of social circumstances," we find no statement whatsoever. In fact, there is barely a word in the entire manual about the nature of schools, neighborhoods, housing, recreational facilities, or other environmental factors which promote healthy development. Only the nuclear family unit is considered as a socializing agent with attention concentrated on the role of mother and father. There is complete silence concerning the nature of the future life circumstances toward which each individual is developing. There is an implicit acceptance of the part that socializing agents will play in preparing individuals for future life roles. Since the definition of the mature personality includes the ability to work, we can safely conclude that any characteristic which seems to foreshadow difficulty in meeting the demands of the adult role as that role is presently understood will be viewed as deviant, and therefore dangerous.

We propose that we accept the view that work is obsolete and that it makes little difference how an individual spends his time, as long as he does not physically hurt others. Let us say that it makes no real difference whether he chooses to spend his time developing skills related to what we now accept as work, whether he develops skills we now classify as leisure activities, or whether he decides to be contemplative. An intellectually oriented child might want to learn to read and write; a motorically oriented child might want to learn to run, to jump, to climb; a socially oriented child might want to spend time playing and talking with others who want to play and talk; while a passive child might well decide to be a spectator. In other words, that behavior which was previously considered deviation, because it contained within it the threat of a continued dependency, may now be considered an acceptable form of variation. Rather than deviation, it now becomes diversity.

The reduced need to commit human energies to making a living creates a situation in which it becomes imperative to encourage and to value a great variety of ways of being. The present time is a period of acute social change and many social institutions must change if they are to be congruent with the way people already are living. There are profound implications, particularly for those institutions concerned with transmitting the essential skills for living in the world.

Since more people are spending more of the life span in formal schooling, it becomes a legitimate question to ask whether people desire to spend that amount of time engaged in tasks set for them by others, or whether there are not other ways in which they would prefer to live.

Even if school is necessary as a preparation for life, then curriculum and methods should emphasize the development of leisure and recreational skills. The capacity for active and passive enjoyment should be developed through the education of the senses and the mind. If boredom is to be avoided, then the capacity for creativity should be released. The ability to construct novelty or to find novelty in the familiar becomes critical. The individual should learn to evaluate what he does and what he experiences, not in terms of external criteria, but in terms of self-satisfaction and the attainment of his own goals. Children are evaluated continually by others on their performance in tasks set by others. We venture to guess that the number of real decisions children make in school about the activities in which they will engage is next to zero. Not only must individuals learn to prepare for a situation where choice and self-evaluation replace the tendency to engage in activities and meet standards set by others, but the criteria of production should change from narrowly academic ones to the achievement of the peak experience (Maslow, 1962).

There is still another issue related to creativity. Since it can be safely predicted that all knowledge rapidly becomes obsolete, it is necessary to realize that each individual will be required to adapt to a number of far-reaching changes in the course of his lifetime. Adaptation to change demands that individuals acquire not facts or the ability to take in passively but active attitudes toward learning. Adaptation to change requires a sense of confidence in one's learning skills. The new should be approached not with dread, but rather with a joyous sense that one will grow by having mastered a challenge. One must learn to feel comfortable with uncertainty and to take chances without feeling that mistakes are irretrievable or disastrous. Short-answer achievement tests are inadequate measures of how well children are prepared "to learn to learn" and therefore are inadequate measures of the schools themselves.

The necessity to encourage and to value a vastly greater variety of ways of being requires a drastic change in concepts of interpersonal relationships. The ability to mind one's own business, to work with mindless concentration upon a simple, repetitive operation alongside other human beings is no longer essential nor sufficient for living in the world. Face-to-face, emotionally stimulating interactions may become much more the social requirement in a world of abundance, while competitive relationships and dominance-subordinance relationships may become less critical in maintaining a social order. The essential skills will be techniques of creating the human environment that encourages growth and pleasure in others. We can add that our current experience in a variety of work settings reveals that interpersonal tensions, competitiveness, rivalries, cliques, jealousies, backbiting, and the like are rampant, with consequent failures in communication and cooperation. The ideal is far from being attained, and the problem may well reflect serious deficiencies in interpersonal competence in a world which has already changed substantially. Little or nothing in classrooms prepares for effective human interaction. Most classroom situations encourage submission (Henry, 1965), are teacher centered (Medley & Mitzel, 1963), thwart curiosity, and do not encourage communication which would promote understanding of psychological and emotional processes in others (Susskind, 1968). In other words, observers of contemporary schools report that the schools are not providing individuals with the skills necessary to make a full life in the world. From that viewpoint, they are contributing to mental health problems.

We have restricted our analysis to schools because our experience is greatest in that area. However, work settings, laws which govern marital and sexual conduct, personal pleasures, the small nuclear family, welfare and mental health services are all changing. In each instance the valence is toward freer choice, toward greater tolerance of different forms of expression of pleasures, and toward a greater sharing of previously restricted functions.

The lessons for the mental health professional seem clear. He cannot permit himself to function as an agent of deviancy control viewing each new development as an alarming manifestation of social pathology. In so doing he promotes social problems by supporting outmoded norms of conduct, thus blocking solutions by retarding the reduction of cultural lag.

Perhaps the following passage from Jane Addams expresses the attitude the social scientist and the mental health professional might adopt toward social change:

> As these overworked girls stream along the street, the rest of us see only the self-conscious walk, the giggling speech, the preposterous clothing. And yet through the huge

hat, the wilderness of bedraggled feathers, the girl announces to the world that she is here. She demands attention to the fact of her existence, she states that she is ready to live, to take her place in the world. The most precious moment in human development is the young creature's assertion that he is unlike any other human being, and has an individual contribution to make to the world. The variation from the established type is at the root of all change, the only possible basis for progress, all that keeps life from growing unprofitably stale and repetitious (Addams, 1909, p. 88).

We suggest that the mental health professional needs to direct his attention toward techniques for reducing cultural lag and toward diagnosing the institutional contributions to problems in living. If our society is now in a period of acute change then history and theory demand that some substantial proportion of mental health professionals direct their attention toward understanding and facilitating concomitant changes. Today then is the time for action; the challenge we face is to turn the concepts we acquired yesterday to the problems we will face tomorrow.

bibliography

Abbott, E., & Breckinridge, S. P. *Truancy and non-attendance in the Chicago schools.* Chicago: University of Chicago Press, 1917.

Abell, A. I. *The urban impact on American Protestantism: 1865–1890.* Cambridge: Harvard University Press, 1943.

Abelson, W. D. *A clinic in the community.* New Haven: Clifford W. Beers Guidance Clinic, Inc., 1966.

Adams, F. P. Personal glimpses. A glimpse of Ben Lindsey justice. *Literary Digest,* April 3, 1915, **50,** 762–766.

Addams, J. *The spirit of youth and the city streets.* New York: Macmillan, 1909.

Addams, J. *Twenty years at Hull House.* New York: Macmillan, 1910.

Addams, J., et al. *The child, the clinic and the court.* New York: New Republic, 1925.

Addams, J. A toast to John Dewey. *Survey* 1929, **63,** 203–204.

Additon, H. *City planning for girls. Soc. Serv. Monogr. No. 5.* Chicago: University of Chicago Press, 1928.

Adler, H. M. *A behavioristic study of delinquency.* Proceedings of forty-sixth annual session of the American Association for the Study of the Feebleminded. St. Louis, May, 1922.

AFL-CIO Department of Research. *Labor looks at automation.* New York: AFL-CIO, 1959.

AFL-CIO Community Services Activities. *The shorter work week and the constructive use of free time.* Proceedings of the Eighth Annual AFL-CIO National Conference on Community Services. New York, 1963.

Albee, G. W. *Mental health manpower trends.* New York: Basic Books, 1959.

Albee, G. W. No magic here. (Review of R. Glasscote, D. Sanders, H. M. Forstenzer and A. R. Foley [Eds.] *The community mental health center: An analysis of existing models.* Washington, D.C.: American Psychiatric Association, 1964). *Contemporary Psychology,* 1965, **10,** 497–498.

Allen, E. A mental hygiene program in grade schools. *Mental Hygiene,* 1929, **13,** 289–297.

Allen, F. H. The Philadelphia Child Guidance Clinic. In L. G. Lowrey and V. Sloane (Eds.) *Orthopsychiatry, 1923–1948. Retrospect and prospect.* New York: American Orthopsychiatric Association, 1948.

Allen, F. L. *Only yesterday.* New York: Bantam Books, 1959.

Atkinson, C., & Maleska, E. T. *The story of education.* New York: Bantam Books, 1964.

Bailyn, B. *Education in the forming of American society.* New York: Vintage Books, 1960.

Barker, L. F. The first ten years of the National Committee for Mental Hygiene, with some comments on its future. *Mental Hygiene,* 1918, **2,** 557–581.

Barnett, H. The beginning of Toynbee Hall. In L. M. Pacey (Ed.) *Readings in the development of settlement work.* New York: Association Press, 1950.

Bazelon, D. T. The paper economy. *Commentary,* September, 1962, **33,** 185–197.

Beard, C. A., & Beard, M. R. *The rise of American civilization.* Vol. II. *The industrial era.* New York: Macmillan, 1927.

Beers, C. W. *A mind that found itself.* Garden City: Doubleday Doran, 1933 (5th rev. ed., 1921).

Beilen, H. Teachers' and clinicians' attitudes toward the behavior problems of children, a reappraisal. In V. Noll & R. Noll (Eds.) *Readings in educational psychology.* New York: Macmillan, 1962.

Bernstein, P. *The lean years: A history of the American worker. 1920–1933.* Baltimore: Penguin Books, 1966.

Bernstein, R. J. *John Dewey.* New York: Washington Square Press, 1967.

Blanton, S. The function of the mental hygiene clinic in the schools and colleges. In J. Addams, et al. *The child, the clinic and the court.* New York: New Republic, 1925.

Blatt, B., & Kaplan, F. *Christmas in purgatory.* Boston: Allyn & Bacon, 1966.

Bordin, R. Emma Hall and the reformatory principle. *Michigan History,* 1964, **48,** 315–332.

Boring, E. G. *A history of experimental psychology.* (2nd ed.) New York: Appleton-Century-Crofts, 1957.

Bourne, R. S. *The Gary Schools.* Boston: Houghton Mifflin, 1916.

Bowen, J. T. The early days of the juvenile court. In J. Addams, et al., *The child, the clinic and the court.* New York: New Republic, 1925.

Brightbill, C. K. *The challenge of leisure.* Englewood Cliffs, N.J.: Prentice-Hall, 1960.

Brill, A. A. The introduction and development of Freud's work in the United States. *Amer. J. Sociol.,* 1939, **45,** 318–325.

Brotemarkle, R. A. (Ed.) *Clinical Psychology. Studies in honor of Lightner Witmer.* Philadelphia: University of Pennsylvania Press, 1931.

Bryant, J. E. A method for determining the extent and causes of retardation in a city school system. *Psychological Clinic,* 1906–1907, **1,** 41–52.

Burgess, E. W. The influence of Sigmund Freud on sociology in the United States. *Amer. J. Sociol.*, 1939, 45, 356–374.

Callahan, D. The quest for social relevance. *Daedalus*, 1967, 96, 151–179.

Campbell, C. M. A city school district and its subnormal children; with a discussion of some social problems involved and suggestions for constructive work. *Mental Hygiene*, 1918, 2, 232–244.

Campbell, C. M. Education and mental hygiene. *Mental Hygiene*, 1919, 3, 398–408.

Caplow, T. *The sociology of work.* New York: McGraw-Hill, 1964.

Carmichael, S., & Hamilton, C. V. *Black power.* New York: Vintage Books, 1967.

Carr, E. H. *What is history?* New York: Alfred A. Knopf, 1963.

Chambers, C. A. Seedtime of reform. *American Social Service and Social Action, 1918–1933.* Ann Arbor: University of Michigan Press, 1967.

Charlesworth, J. C. (Ed.) *Leisure in America: Blessing or curse.* Monograph No. 4, American Academy of Political and Social Science, 1964.

Children's Bureau. Juvenile Court Statistics, 1963. *Children's Bureau Statistical Series*, No. 79, Washington, D.C.: U.S. Department of Health, Education and Welfare, 1964.

Clark, B. R. Sociology of Education. In R. L. Faris (Ed.) *Handbook of Modern Sociology:* Chicago: Rand McNally, 1964.

Cohen, N. E. *Social work in the American tradition.* New York: Holt, Rinehart & Winston 1958.

Coit, S. *Neighborhood guilds. An instrument of social reform.* London: Swan Sonnenschein, 1891.

Coleman, J. S., Campbell, E. Q., Hobson, C. J., McPartland, J., Mood, A. M., Weinfeld, F. D., & York, R. L. *Equality of educational opportunity.* Supt. Documents, Catalog No. FS 5.238:38001. Washington, D.C.: U.S. Government Printing Office, 1966.

Colorado Humane Society. *Child and animal protection.* Sept. 1910, 3, No. 26. (Unsigned article.)

Committee of Syracuse Board of Education to investigate the school system of Gary, Inc. *The Gary System.* Syracuse: C. W. Bardeen, 1915.

Commonwealth Fund. *Fourth Annual Report. 1921–1922.* New York: Commonwealth Fund, 1922.

Commonwealth Fund. *Historical Sketch. 1918–1962.* New York: Harkness House, 1963.

Community Progress, Inc. *The human story.* New Haven: CPI, 1966.

Cornman, O. P. The retardation of the pupils of five city school systems. *Psychological Clinic*, 1906–1907, 1, 245–257.

Coulter, E. K. *The children in the shadow.* New York: McBride, Nast, 1913.

Courtis, S. A. *Measurement of classroom products.* New York: General Education Board, 1919.

Cox, H. G. The "new breed" in American churches: Sources of social activism in American religion. *Daedalus*, 1967, 96, 135–150.

Cremin, L. A. *The transformation of the school.* New York: Vintage Books, 1964.

Cross, W. L. (Ed.) *Twenty-five years after: Sidelights on the mental hygiene movement and its founder.* New York: Doubleday, Doran, 1934.

Cumming, E., & Cumming, J. *Closed ranks.* Cambridge: Harvard University Press, 1957.

Cumming, J., & Cumming, E. On the stigma of mental illness. *Community Mental Health Journal,* 1965, **1,** 135–143.

Curti, M. *The growth of American thought.* New York: Harper, 1951.

Davie, M. *Sumner today: Selected essays of William Graham Sumner.* New Haven: Yale University Press, 1940.

Davis, A. F. *Spearheads for reform: The social settlements and the progressive movement, 1890–1914.* Unpublished Ph.D. thesis, University of Wisconsin, 1959. (University Microfilms 59-5758)

DeGrazia, S. *Of time, work and leisure.* New York: Twentieth Century Fund, 1962.

Denver Christian Citizenship Union. *The Civic Review. Quarterly Bulletin,* 1910, **3,** 3–9.

Devereux, H. T. Report of a year's work on defectives in a public school. *Psychological Clinic,* 1909–1910, **3,** 45–48.

Dewey, J. *My pedagogic creed.* G. L. Kellogg, 1897.

Dewey, J., & Dewey, E. *Schools of tomorrow.* New York: E. P. Dutton, 1915.

Dollard, J. *Caste and class in a Southern town.* New York: Doubleday, 1957.

Duffus, R. L. *Lillian Wald: Neighbor and crusader.* New York: Macmillan, 1938.

Dummer, E. S. Life in relation to time. In L. G. Lowrey & V. Sloane (Eds.) *Orthopsychiatry, 1923–1948. Retrospect and prospect.* New York: American Orthopsychiatric Association, 1948.

Eels, K., Davis, A., Havighurst, R. J., Herrick, V. E., & Tyler, R. M. *Intelligence and cultural differences.* Chicago: University of Chicago Press, 1951.

Eliot, T. D. *The juvenile court and the community.* New York: Macmillan, 1914.

Eysenck, H. J. The effects of psychotherapy: An evaluation. *J. Consult. Psychol.,* 1952, **16,** 319–324.

Eysenck, H. J. The effects of psychotherapy. In H. J. Eysenck (Ed.) *Handbook of abnormal psychology.* New York: Basic Books, 1961.

Flexner, A., & Bachman, F. P. *The Gary schools: A general account.* New York: General Education Board, 1918.

Flexner, A. *I remember.* New York: Simon & Schuster, 1940.

Flexner, A. Is social work a profession? In R. E. Pumphrey & M. W. Pumphrey (Eds.) *The heritage of American social work.* New York: Columbia University Press, 1961.

Flexner, E. *Century of struggle.* Cambridge: Belknap Press, 1966.

Freeman, H. F. University settlement. In R. E. Pumphrey & M. W. Pumphrey (Eds.) *The heritage of American social work.* New York: Columbia University Press, 1961.

French, L. M. *Psychiatric social work.* New York: The Commonwealth Fund, 1940.

Freud, S. *Civilization and its discontents.* London: Hogarth Press, 1930.

Freud, S. Three contributions to the theory of sex. *In Basic Writings of Sigmund Freud.* New York: Modern Library, 1938.

Freud, S. Instincts and their vicissitudes. *Collected Papers.* Vol. IV. New York: Basic Books, 1959.

Furman, S. S. Suggestions for refocusing child guidance clinics. *Children,* 1965, **12**, 140–144.

Furman, S. S., Sweat, L. G., & Crocetti, G. M. Social class factors in the flow of children to outpatient psychiatric facilities. *Amer. J. of Publ. Hlth.,* 1965, **55**, 385–392.

Galbraith, J. K. *The affluent society.* New York: Mentor Books, 1958.

George, H. *Progress and poverty.* New York: Doubleday & McClure, 1879.

Gesell, A. *Infancy and human growth.* New York: Macmillan, 1928.

Glazer, N., & Moynihan, D. P. *Beyond the melting pot.* Cambridge: MIT Press, 1963.

Glueck, B. Special preparation of the psychiatric social worker. *Mental Hygiene,* 1919, **3**, 409–419.

Goffman, E. *Asylums.* New York: Doubleday, 1961.

Goffman, E. *Stigma: Notes on the management of a spoiled identity.* Englewood Cliffs, N.J.: Prentice-Hall, 1963.

Gold, M. *Jews without money.* New York: Liveright, 1930.

Goldhamer, H., & Marshall, A. W. *Psychosis and civilization: Two studies in the frequency of mental disease.* Glencoe, Ill.: The Free Press, 1953.

Goldman, E. F. *Rendezvous with destiny.* New York: Vintage Books, 1956.

Goren, A. A. *The New York Kehillah. 1908–1922.* Unpublished doctoral thesis. Columbia University, 1966.

Gouldner, A. W. The sociologist as partisan: Sociology and the welfare state. *Amer. Sociologist,* 1968, **3**, 103–116.

Grant, Q. A. R., & Stringer, L. A. Design for a new orthopsychiatric discipline. *Amer. J. Orthopsychiat.,* 1964, **34**, 722–729.

Grob, G. N. *The state and the mentally ill.* Durham: The University of North Carolina Press, 1966.

Group for the Advancement of Psychiatry. *Psychopathological disorders in childhood: Theoretical considerations and a proposed classification.* New York: Group for the Advancement of Psychiatry, 1966.

Hall, G. S. *Life and confessions of a psychologist.* New York: D. Appleton, 1923.

Handlin, O. *The uprooted.* New York: Grosset & Dunlap, 1951.

Handlin, O. *Immigration as a factor in American history.* Englewood Cliffs, N.J.: Prentice-Hall, 1959.

Hapgood, H. *The spirit of the ghetto.* Cambridge: Belknap Press, 1967.

Haring, N. G., & Phillips, E. L. *Educating emotionally disturbed children.* New York: McGraw-Hill, 1962.

Harrison, S. I., McDermott, J. F., Wilson, P. T., & Schrager, J. Social class and mental illness in children: Choice of treatment. *Arch. General Psychiat.,* 1965, **13**, 411–417.

Hays, S. P. *The response to industrialism.* Chicago: University of Chicago Press, 1957.

Healy, W. *The individual delinquent*. Boston: Little, Brown, 1915.

Healy, W., & Bronner, A. F. An outline for institutional education and treatment of young offenders. *J. Educ. Psychol.*, 1915, **6**, 301–316.

Healy, W. The psychology of the situation: A fundamental for understanding and treatment of delinquency and crime. In J. Addams, et al., *The child, the clinic and the court*. New York: New Republic, 1925.

Healy, W., & Bronner, A. F. *Delinquents and criminals: Their making and unmaking*. New York: Macmillan, 1926.

Healy, W., & Healy, M. T. *Pathological lying, accusation, and swindling*. Criminal Science Monograph No. 1. Boston: Little, Brown, 1926.

Healy, W., Bronner, A. F., & Bowers, A. M. *The structure and meaning of psychoanalysis*. New York: Knopf, 1931.

Healy, W., & Bronner, A. F. The child guidance clinic: Birth and growth of an idea. In L. G. Lowrey & V. Sloane (Eds.) *Orthopsychiatry, 1923–1948. Retrospect and Prospect*. New York: American Orthopsychiatric Association, 1948, pp. 14–49.

Heilman, J. D. The need for special classes in the public schools. *Psychological Clinic, 1906–1907*, **1**, 104–114.

Henderson, N. *Visiting teachers: The work of visiting teachers employed by the Public Education Society, 1910–1911*. New York: Public Education Society, 1910–1911.

Henry, J. *Culture against man*. New York: Random House, 1965.

Hoffman, C. W. Organization of family courts with special reference to the juvenile court. In J. Addams, et al. *The child, the clinic and the court*. New York: New Republic, 1925.

Hofstadter, R. *Social Darwinism in American thought*. Rev. ed. Boston: The Beacon Press, 1955.

Holden, A. C. *The settlement idea: A vision of social justice*. New York: Macmillan, 1922.

Hollingshead, A. B. *Elmtown's youth*. New York: Wiley, 1949.

Hollingshead, A. B., & Redlich, F. C. *Social class and mental illness*. New York: Wiley, 1958.

Hopkins, C. H. *The rise of the social gospel in American Protestantism, 1865–1915*. New Haven: Yale University Press, 1940.

International Prison Commission. *Children's Courts in the United States: Their origin, development, and results*. Washington, D.C.: Government Printing Office, 1904.

James, H. (Ed.) *The letters of William James*. 2 vols. Boston: Little, Brown, 1926.

James, W. *Talks to teachers*. New York: Holt, 1899.

Jarrett, M. C. Psychiatric social work. *Mental Hygiene*, 1918, **2**, 283-290.

Johnson, H. M. *The visiting teacher in New York City*. New York: Public Education Association of the City of New York, 1916.

Joint Commission on Mental Illness and Health. *Action for mental health*. New York: Basic Books, 1961.

Kanner, L. Emotionally disturbed children: A historical review. *Child Development*, 1962, **33**, 97–102.

Kanner, L. *A history of the care and study of the mentally retarded.* Springfield, Ill.: Charles C. Thomas, 1964.

Kessen, W. *The child.* New York: Wiley, 1965.

Key, E. *Century of the child.* New York: Putnam, 1909.

Klein, V. *The feminine character.* New York: International Universities Press, 1946.

Knobloch, H., & Pasamanick, B. Some thoughts on the inheritance of intelligence. *Amer. J. Orthopsychiat.,* 1961, 31, 454–473.

Lasch, C. (Ed.) *The social thought of Jane Addams.* Indianapolis: Bobbs Merrill, 1965.

Lasch, C. *The new radicalism in America, 1889–1963: The intellectual as a social type.* New York: Vintage Books, 1967.

Lathrop, J. C. The background of the juvenile court in Illinois. In J. Addams, et al., *The child, the clinic and the court.* New York: New Republic, 1925.

Lee, P. R., and Kenworthy, M. E. *Mental hygiene and social work.* New York: Commonwealth Fund, Division of Publications, 1929.

Leighton, D. C., Harding, J. S., Macklin, D. B., Macmillan, A. M., & Leighton, A. H. *The character of danger: Psychiatric symptoms in selected communities.* New York: Basic Books, 1963.

Levine, D., & Levine, Z. Political activity in the social settlements. Unpublished Science Fair Study Report. Hamden, Connecticut. April, 1967.

Levine, M., & Levine, A. Social change and psychopathology: Some derivations from *"Civilization and its Discontents."* In G. D. Goldman and D. N. Milman (Eds.) *The contributions of psychoanalysis to community psychology.* Springfield, Ill.: Charles C. Thomas. (In press.)

Levitt, E. E. The results of psychotherapy with children: An evaluation. *J. consult. Psychol.,* 1957, 21, 189–196.

Levitt, E. E., Beiser, H. R., & Robertson, R. E. A follow-up evaluation of cases treated at a community guidance clinic. *Amer. J. Orthopsychiat.,* 1959, 29, 337–349

Levy, D. M. Critical evaluation of the present state of child psychiatry. *Amer. J. Psychiat.,* 1952, 108, 481–494.

Lindsey, B. B. The reformation of juvenile delinquents through the juvenile court. Paper read before the National Conference of Charities and Corrections, 30th Annual Meeting, Atlanta, 1903.

Lindsey, B. B. *Juvenile Court of Denver. The problem of the children and how the state of Colorado cares for them.* Denver: Merchants Publishing Company, 1904.

Lindsey, B. B. Colorado's contribution to the juvenile court. In J. Addams, et al., *The child, the clinic and the court.* New York: New Republic, 1925.

Lindsey, B. B. The juvenile court of the future. *Annual report and proceedings of the National Probation Association,* 1925.

Lindsey, B. B., & Borough, R. *The dangerous life.* New York: Liveright, 1931.

Lindsey, B. B., & Evans, W. *The revolt of modern youth.* New York: Boni & Liveright, 1925.

Lindsey, B. B., & O'Higgins, H. J. *The beast.* New York: Doubleday, Page, 1910.

Linn, J. W. *Jane Addams: A biography.* New York: D. Appleton-Century, 1935.

Loring, E. R. Some adaptive difficulties found in school children. *Mental Hygiene*, 1920, **4**, 330–363.

Lowrey, L. G., & Smith, G. *The institute for child guidance. 1927–1933.* New York: Commonwealth Fund, 1933.

Lowrey, L. G. Orthopsychiatric treatment. In Lowrey, L. G., & Sloane, V. (Eds.) *Orthopsychiatry, 1923–1948. Retrospect and prospect.* New York: American Orthopsychiatric Association, 1948.

Lukas, A. Jewish federation: 50 rewarding years of diverse philanthropy. *The New York Times*, Sept. 28, 1967.

Lynd, R. S., & Lynd, H. M. *Middletown.* New York: Harcourt Brace, 1929.

Lynd, S. Jane Addams and the radical impulse. *Commentary*, 1961, **32**, 54–59.

Machlup, F. *The production and distribution of knowledge in the United States.* Princeton: Princeton University Press, 1962.

Mack, J. W. The chancery procedure in the juvenile court. In J. Addams, et al. *The child, the clinic and the court.* New York: New Republic, 1925.

Maslow, A. H. *Toward a psychology of being.* Princeton: D. Van Nostrand, 1962.

May, E. *The wasted Americans.* New York: Signet Books, 1964.

Medley, D. M., & Mitzel, H. E. Measuring classroom behavior by systematic observation. In N. L. Gage (Ed.) *Handbook of research on teaching.* Chicago: Rand McNally, 1963.

Meehl, P. E. *Clinical versus statistical prediction.* Minneapolis: University of Minnesota Press, 1954.

Meehl, P. E. The cognitive activity of the clinician. *Amer. Psychologist*, 1960, **15**, 19–27.

Mensh, I. N. *Clinical psychology: Science and profession.* New York: Macmillan, 1966.

Miller, K. D., & Miller, E. P. *The people are the city.* New York: Macmillan, 1962.

Miner, M. E. *Slavery of prostitution.* New York: Macmillan, 1916.

Monroe, P. (Ed.) *A cyclopedia of education.* New York: Macmillan, 1911.

Montessori, M. *The Montessori method.* New York: Schocken Books, 1964.

Moynihan, D. P. *The Negro family: The case for national action.* Washington, D.C.: Office of Policy Planning and Research, U.S. Department of Labor, 1965.

Murstein, B. I. *Theory and research in projective techniques.* New York: Wiley, 1963.

Myers, J. K., & Schaffer, L. Social stratification and psychiatric practice: A study of an out-patient clinic. In E. Gartly Jaco (Ed.) *Patients, Physicians and Illness.* Glencoe, Ill.: The Free Press, 1958. pp. 501–506.

National Association of Visiting Teachers and Home and School Visitors. *The visiting teacher in the US.* Public Education Association of New York: New York, 1921.

Neilson, W. A. The Smith College experiment in training for psychiatric social work. *Mental Hygiene,* 1919, 3, 59–64.

Newman, R. G. *Psychological consultation in the schools: A catalyst for learning.* New York: Basic Books, 1967.

Oberndorf, C. P. *A history of psychoanalysis in America.* New York: Grune & Stratton, 1953.

Oppenheimer, J. J. *The visiting teacher movement, with special reference to administrative relationships.* New York: Joint Committee on Preventing Delinquency, 1925.

Parker, S. W. Orthogenic cases. XII. A study of the interplay of personality. *The Psychological Clinic,* 1917–1918, 11, 97–111; 129–141; 157-178.

Pastore, N. *The nature-nurture controversy.* New York: Kings Crown Press, 1949.

Personal Glimpses. Why children trust Ben Lindsey. *Literary Digest,* 1915, Dec. 25, 50, 1506–1508.

Peterson, J. *Early conceptions and tests of intelligence.* Yonkers: World Book, 1926.

Phillips, D. L. Identification of mental illness. Its consequences for rejection. *Commun. Mentl. Hlth. J.,* 1967, 3, 262–266.

Pierce, F. The Federal government—the great almoner? In R. E. Pumphrey & M. W. Pumphrey (Eds.) *The heritage of American social work.* New York: Columbia University Press, 1961, pp. 132–134.

Polier, J. W. *A view from the bench: The Juvenile Court.* New York: National Council on Crime and Delinquency, 1964.

Polsky, H. W. *Cottage six.* New York: Russell Sage Foundation, 1962.

Powdermaker, H. *Stranger and friend.* New York: W. W. Norton, 1966.

Pumphrey, R. E., & Pumphrey, M. W. (Eds.) *The heritage of American social work.* New York: Columbia University Press, 1961.

Raine, W. M. How Judge Lindsey handles his boys. *Ladies Home Journal,* May, 1907.

Rainwater, L. Crucible of identity: The Negro lower-class family. *Daedalus,* Winter, 1966.

Redl, F. *When we deal with children.* New York: The Free Press, 1966.

Redl, F., & Wineman, D. *Children who hate.* New York: The Free Press, 1951.

Reiss, B. F. & Brandt, L. W. What happens to applicants for psychotherapy? *Commun. Mentl. Hlth. J.,* 1965, 1, 175–180.

Report of the City Superintendent of Schools. New York, 1913–1914.

Report of the Hartford Vice Commission. Hartford, 1913.

Report of the Immigration Commission on the Importation and Harboring of Women for Immoral purposes. Senate Document, 196, 1909, 23.

Report of the International Society for the Rescue of Jewish Women and Children. New York, 1927.

Report of the Juvenile Court—City and County of Denver, Nov. 1, 1908–Nov. 1, 1909.

Report of Juvenile Court—City and County of Denver, Nov. 1, 1909–Oct. 31, 1910.

Report of Juvenile Division of County Court. Arapahoe County, Jan. 1901–July, 1902.

Report of the Moral Survey Committee on the Social Evil. Syracuse, 1913.

Richmond, M. E. Good spirit and earnestness. In R. E. Pumphrey & M. W. Pumphrey (Eds.) *The heritage of American social work.* New York: Columbia University Press, 1961.

Richmond, M. E. *Social diagnosis.* New York: Free Press, 1965.

Rickers-Ovsiankina, M. A. (Ed.) *Rorschach psychology.* New York: Wiley, 1960.

Ridenour, N. Mental health education. In L. G. Lowrey & V. Sloane (Eds.) *Orthopsychiatry, 1923–1948: Retrospect and prospect.* New York: American Orthopsychiatric Association, 1948.

Riis, J. *The battle with the slums.* New York: Macmillan, 1902.

Riis, J. *How the other half lives.* New York: Charles Scribner's, 1917.

Riordan, W. L. *Plunkitt of Tammany Hall.* New York: McClure Phillips, 1905.

Roback, A. A. *A history of American psychology.* New York: Collier Books, 1964.

Roback, A. A. *History of psychology and psychiatry.* New York: Citadel Press, 1964.

Robison, S. M. A study of delinquency among Jewish children in New York City. In M. Sklare (Ed.) *The Jews: Social patterns of an American group.* New York: Free Press, 1958.

Rosenblum, G., & Ottenstein, D. From child guidance to community mental health. *Commun. Mntl. Hlth. J.,* 1965, 1, 276–283.

Sarason, S. B. *Psychological problems in mental deficiency.* 3rd Ed. New York: Harper & Row, 1958.

Sarason, S. B., & Doris, J. *Psychological problems in mental deficiency.* 4th Ed. New York: Harper & Row, 1969.

Sarason, S. B., Levine, M., Goldenberg, I. I., Cherlin, D. L., & Bennett, E. M. *Psychology in community settings: Clinical, educational, vocational, social aspects.* New York: Wiley, 1966.

Sarnoff, D. The social impact of computers. Address to the American Bankers Association, National Automation Conference. New York World's Fair, July, 1964.

Sayles, M. B. *Three problem children: Narratives from the case records of a child guidance clinic.* New York: Joint Committee on Methods of Preventing Delinquency, 1926.

Scheff, T. S. *Being mentally ill: A sociological theory.* New York: Aldine, 1966.

Schlesinger, A. M. *The Age of Roosevelt: The crisis of the old order, 1919–1933.* Boston: Houghton Mifflin, 1957.

Schumacher, H. C. The Cleveland Guidance Center. In L. G. Lowrey &

V. Sloane (Eds.) *Orthopsychiatry 1923–1948: Retrospect and prospect.* New York: American Orthopsychiatric Association, 1948.

Sexton, P. C. *Education and income.* New York: Viking Press, 1961.

Shakow, D. Clinical psychology: An evaluation. In L. G. Lowrey & V. Sloane (Eds.) *Orthopsychiatry 1923–1948: Retrospect and prospect.* New York: American Orthopsychiatric Association, 1948.

Smith, T. L. The development of psychological clinics in the United States. *Pedagogical Seminary,* 1914, **21**, 143–153.

Smuts, R. *Women and work in America.* New York: Columbia University Press, 1959.

Southard, E. E. Notes on public institutional work in mental prophylaxis. *J. A. M. A.,* 1914, **63**, 1898–1903.

Southard, E. E. Mental hygiene and social work: Notes on a course in social psychiatry for social workers. *Mental Hygiene,* 1918, **2**, 395–406.

Southard, E. E., & Jarrett, M. C. *The kingdom of evils.* New York: Macmillan, 1922.

Spaulding, E., III. The course in social psychiatry. *Mental Hygiene,* 1918, **2**, 586–589.

Spencer, H. *The study of sociology.* New York: D. Appleton, 1873.

Srole, L., Langner, T. S., Michael, S. T., Opler, M. K., & Rennie, T. A. C. *Mental health in the metropolis: The midtown Manhattan study.* New York: McGraw-Hill, 1962.

Steffens, L. *The shame of the cities.* New York: McClure Phillips, 1904.

Steffens, L. *Upbuilders.* New York: Doubleday, Page, 1909.

Steffens, L. *The autobiography of Lincoln Steffens.* New York: Harcourt Brace, 1931.

Stein, H. D. Jewish social work in the United States: 1920–1955. In M. Sklare (Ed.) *The Jews: Social patterns of an American group.* New York: Free Press, 1958.

Stevenson, G. S., & Smith, G. *Child guidance clinics: A quarter century of development.* New York: Commonwealth Fund, 1934.

Stevenson, G. S. The development of extra-mural psychiatry in the United States. *Amer. J. Psychiat.,* 1944, **100**, 147–150.

Stevenson, G. S. Child guidance and the National Committee for mental hygiene. In L. G. Lowrey & V. Sloane (Eds.) *Orthopsychiatry 1923–1948: Retrospect and prospect.* New York: American Orthopsychiatric Association, 1948.

Sullivan, H. S. *The fusion of psychiatry and social science.* New York: W. W. Norton, 1964. (Introduction by Helen Swick Perry.)

Sumner, W. G. *What social classes owe to each other.* New York: Harper's, 1883.

Susskind, E. The role of questions in the elementary school classroom. In F. Kaplan & S. B. Sarason (Eds.) *Collected papers of the Psycho-Educational Clinic.* (In press.)

Sutherland, E. H., & Cressey, D. R. *Principles of criminology.* (6th Ed.) Philadelphia: J. B. Lippincott, 1960.

Taylor, J. S. A report on the Gary experiment in New York. *Educational Review*, New York, 1916, pp. 8–28.

Theobald, R. *The challenge of abundance.* New York: Mentor Books, 1961.

Thomas, W. I., & Thomas, D. S. *The child in America.* New York: Alfred A. Knopf, 1928.

Tuckman, J., & Lavell, M. Attrition in psychiatric clinics for children. *Public Health Reports, Public Health Service*, 1959, **74**, 309–315.

Van Sickle, J. H., Witmer, L., & Ayres, L. P. Provision for exceptional children in public schools. *U.S. Bureau of Education Bulletin*, 1911, No. 14, Whole No. 461.

Veroff, J., Feld, S., & Gurin, G. *Americans view their mental health.* New York: Basic Books, 1960.

Vollmer, H. The juvenile court. Paper read before Contemporary Club, Davenport, Iowa, 1906.

Wald, L. *The home on Henry Street.* New York: Holt, 1915.

Waller, W. *The sociology of teaching.* New York: John Wiley, 1932.

Walsh, J. L., & Elling, R. H. Professionalism and the poor: Structural effects and professional behavior. *J. Hlth. & Social. Behav.*, 1968, **9**, 16–28.

Watson, J. B. *Psychological care of infant and child.* New York: W. W. Norton, 1928.

Watson, R. I. A brief history of clinical psychology. *Psychol. Bull.*, 1953, **50**, 321–346.

Weber, M. *The theory of social and economic organization.* Glencoe, Ill.: Free Press, 1964.

White, M. A., & Harris, M. W. *The school psychologist.* New York: Harper, 1961.

White, R. C. Social workers in society: Some further evidence. *Soc. Work J.*, 1953, **34**, 161–164.

Wickman, E. K. *Children's behavior and teachers' attitudes.* New York: Commonwealth Fund Division of Publications, 1928.

Wilensky, H. L., & Lebeaux, C. N. *Industrial society and social welfare.* New York: Free Press, 1965.

Wirt, W. A. *Newer ideals in education. The complete use of the school plant.* Philadelphia: Public Education Association, 1912.

Wirtz, W. Address to the annual Citizens Action Commission Meeting, New Haven, Conn., Feb., 1964. *Community Progress, 1964*, **1**, No. 3.

Witmer, H. L., & students. The outcome of treatment in a child guidance clinic. *Smith College Studies in Social Work*, 1933, **4**.

Witmer, H. L. *Psychiatric clinics for children.* New York: Commonwealth Fund, 1940.

Witmer, L. The organization of practical work in psychology. *Psychol. Rev.*, 1897, **4**, 116–117.

Witmer, L. *Analytical psychology.* Boston: Ginn, 1902.

Witmer, L. Clinical psychology. *Psychological Clinic*, 1906–1907, **1**, 1–9.

Witmer, L. The hospital school. *Psychological Clinic*, 1908–1909, **2**, 138–146.

Witmer, L. Retardation through neglect in children of the rich. *Psychological Clinic*, 1908–1909, **2**, 157–174.

Witmer, L. Retrospect and prospect: An editorial. *Psychological Clinic*, 1908–1909, **2**, 1–4.

Witmer, L. The treatment and cure of a case of mental and moral defiency. *The Psychological Clinic*, 1908–1909, **2**, 153–179.

Witmer, L. *The special class for backward children.* Philadelphia: Psychological Clinic Press, 1911.

Witmer, L. The exceptional child: At home and in school. In *University lectures delivered by Members of the Faculty in the Free Public Lecture Course, 1913–1914.* Philadelphia: University of Pennsylvania Press, 1915, pp. 534–555.

Witmer, L. Diagnostic education: An education for the fortunate few. *The Psychological Clinic*, 1917–1918, **11**, 69–78.

Witmer, L. Orthogenic Cases, XIV—Don: A curable case of arrested development due to a fear psychosis, the result of shock in a three-year-old infant. *Psychological Clinic*, 1919–1920, **13**, 97-111.

Witmer, L. Psychological diagnosis and the psychonomic orientation of analytic science. An epitome. In R. A. Brotemarkle (Ed.) *Clinical Psychology. Studies in honor of Lightner Witmer.* Philadelphia: University of Pennsylvania Press, 1931.

Witty, P. A., & Theman, V. The psycho-educational clinic. *J. Appl. Psychol.*, 1934, **18**, 369–392.

Woods, R. A. *English social movements.* New York: Charles Scribner's, 1891.

Woods, R. A. *The city wilderness: A settlement study.* Boston: Houghton Mifflin, 1898.

Woods, R. A. Social work: A new profession. *Charities*, 1906, **15**, 469–476.

Woods, R. A., & Kennedy, A. J. *Handbook of settlements.* New York: Russell Sage Foundation Charities Publication Committee, 1911.

Woods, R. A., & Kennedy, A. J. *The settlement horizon: A national estimate.* New York: Russell Sage Foundation, 1922.

Zubin, J., Eron, L. D., & Schumer, F. *An experimental approach to projective techniques.* New York: John Wiley, 1965.

name index

subject index

312

DATE DUE

GAYLORD

PRINTED IN U.S.A.